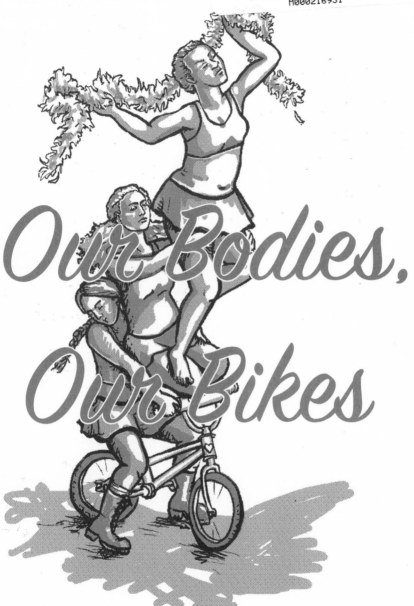

Our Bodies, Our Bikes

OUR BODIES, OUR BIKES

Edited by Elly Blue & April Streeter

Final editorial content © Elly Blue and April Streeter, 2015
This edition © Elly Blue Publishing, an imprint of Microcosm Publishing, 2015
First printing, November 15, 2015
All work remains the property of the original creators.
Made in the USA

ISBN 978-1-62106-895-2

Microcosm Publishing
2752 N Williams Ave.
Portland, OR 97227
TakingTheLane.com
MicrocosmPublishing.com

Cover illustration by Katura Reynolds
Designed by Joe Biel

We have huge admiration for but no affiliation with *Our Bodies, Ourselves* or the Boston Women's Health Project. Go buy that book too, please.

This book collects many voices, mostly women, talking about and illustrating their experience at the intersection of bicycling and gender. None of us are doctors and we don't intend to give you medical advice. Likewise, we don't advocate doing anything that isn't legal where you are or safe by your own judgment. Please enjoy the book and go out and do what's right for you.

"Cycles of Anxiety" was funded by a small grant from the Abortion Conversation Project.

Some of this content has been published previously in an edited form:
Kate Berube's line illustrations appeared in Taking the Lane #2 (*Revolutions*)

"Your Vulva," "My Butt," "BikeSexual" and the accompanying illustration, "Sex Goddess," "How to Be Fast," and "Biking to the Birth Center" appeared in Taking the Lane #5 (*Our Bodies, Our Bikes*), "I See You Baby" appeared in Taking the Lane #6 (*Lines on the Map*)

"When a Sexy M.F. Sneaks up on Your February Morning," "Why it is Great to Date a Cyclist" and Matt Queen's illustrations appeared in Taking the Lane #7 (*BikeSexuality*)

"After the Fact" and "Joining my Son's World" appeared in Taking the Lane #8 (*Childhood*)

A version of "The Bike Test" appeared on TakingtheLane.com

A version of "Cycling up an Appetite" appeared on LovelyBicycle.com

A version of "My Bicycle is my Second Doctor" appeared in The Rivendell Reader #15

"Sausage Party" originally appeared on Bikeyface.com

All content used with enthusiastic permission.

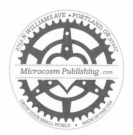

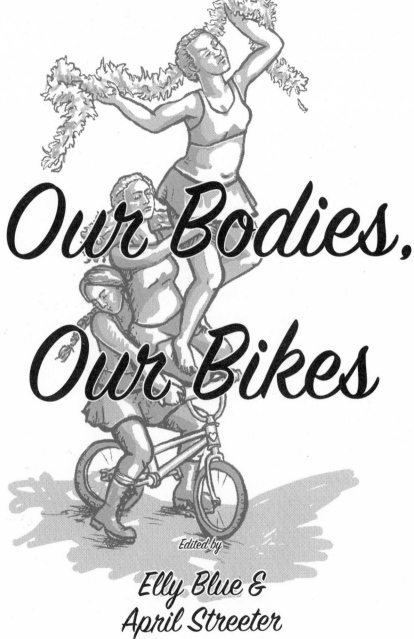

Our Bodies, Our Bikes

Edited by

Elly Blue &
April Streeter

Table of

Introduction 7
Knowledge is Power 10
    The Triple Threat — Samantha Brennan 13
    The Bike Test —Elly Blue 18
Interlude: I See You, Baby — Cecily Walker 23
Being in Our Bodies 24
    On Your Left—Adrian M. Lipscombe 27
    My Butt — Nickey Robare 30
    Cycling Up an Appetite — Constance Winters 32
    Obesity is a Bogeyman — Heidi Guenin 35
Interlude: Biking the Transition — Nathan Ezekiel 38
Safety 40
    The Aha Moment — Echo Rivera 43
    Everything You Want to Know about Biking Safety — Alex Baca and
    Bec Rindler 47
Clothes 50
    Pedaling and Professional Attire — Constance Winters 53
    Dress for Success on the Bike — Janet LaFleur 58
    Every Season — Elly Blue 60
Vulva 62
    How to Make Your Butt Happy — April Streeter 66
    Your Vulva — Elly Blue and Caroline Paquette, RN retired, BSN 70
    The Cuntraption — Adriane Ackerman 75
Menstruation 80
    Biking and Bleeding — Elly Blue 83
    Sustainable Cycles — Rachel Horn 85
Hot Stuff 88
    Sex Goddess on Two Wheels — Jaymi Tharp 91
    Why it's Great to Date a Cyclist — Anonymous 93
    Divorce by Bike — Josie Smith 97
    When a Sexy M.F. Sneaks up on Your February Morning — Rhienna
Renée Guedry 99

Contents

Childbearing 102

    Biking to the Birth Center — Katie Proctor 107

    Biking Towards VBAC — Dena Driscoll 110

    After the Fact — Katura Reynolds 112

Our Bodies, Our Choice 116

    Cycles of Anxiety — Constance Winters 119

    Apologies to Margaret Sanger — K.I. Hope 124

    True Story — C.E. Snow 126

Interlude: Bike Patch — Katie Monroe 128

Menopause 130

    Aging by Bicycle — Susanne Wright 133

    Biking up to the Pause — Elly Blue interviews Beth Hamon ... 136

Interlude: Joining My Son's World — Kathleen Youell ... 140

Sickness and Health 142

    Wheeling — Parisa Emam 145

    You're Too Pretty to be Disabled — Halley Weaver ... 147

    Cars Did This to Me — Lisa Sagrati 150

    Every Breath — Jacqueline A. Gross 156

    My Bicycle is my Second Doctor — Beth Hamon 159

    Bike-Ability — Sarah Rebolloso McCullough 162

    The Physical and Mental Victories of Cycling — Kristin Eagle ... 165

    A License to Bike — Synthia Nicole 167

Interlude: Clearing My Mind—Chelle D. 170

Sports 172

    Equal Pay for Equal Work — Julie Gourinchas 175

    Ass Nebula — Kirsten Rudberg 178

    How to be Fast — Lindsay Kandra 181

    Secrets of Cycling Superpowers — Emily June Street ... 184

Postlude 189

Contributors 190

ILLUSTRATION INDEX

Sausage Festival — Bikeyface 17

Diagram — Keihly Moore 46

Self-Portrait in Professional Attire — Constance Winters 53

Selle Anatomica — Reb Rowe 65

A Lady's Liberators — Reb Rowe 74

Cuntraption in Action — Dabe Alan 77

All Hail the Cuntraption — Dabe Alan 78

Biking Grandma — Suzi Hunt 79

Sustainable Cycles logo 86

Interlude: Bike-By Herbalism — Kelli Refer 87

Picnic Cuddle — Kate Berube 95

I Kissed Ilaria — Matt Queen 96

Burlesque — Matt Queen 101

Venus — W. D. Smith 106

Family — Holly Kvalheim 109

Toddler — Kate Berube 115

Florence — Matt Queen 123

Girls Bike PHL Patch — courtesy of Katie Monroe 128

Butterflies — W.D. Smith 149

The Advertisement — Matt Queen 161

Synthia Nicole — Aaron Poliwoda 167

Girl — Holly Kvalheim 169

Yo Polo — Reb Rowe 177

Grrrls to the Front — Reb Rowe 180

Pilates Poses — Emily June Street 184

Feminists Against Freeways logo — Joe Biel 188

INTRODUCTION

Elly Blue & April Streeter

Why this book?

Here in the United States, we are in the midst of a massive, ongoing public health crisis, with impacts both personal and political. Increasingly, people are taking to two wheels in response. We are using bicycles, bike infrastructure, and pedal-powered community movements as a sort of thread to stitch up the broken parts of our lives, landscapes, and communities.

Of course, as bicycling grows into a national pastime and an increasingly mainstream mode of transportation, the same debates and narratives are turning up in bike communities as are raging in other places—about race, and class, and, of course, gender.

Meanwhile, we are also in the middle of what often feels like a national family dinner table argument about women's rights and the role and meaning of gender in our society and economy. Who should do what work, at home and for pay? Who should be responsible for children? How should a person's decision to have children—or not to do so—affect the other aspects of their lives? The banter often gets silly, but the consequences are very heavy.

On the surface, gender issues have nothing to do with the discourse about cycling (it's great for your health, the economy, and the planet!) that we are used to hearing. But on a deeper level, every aspect of the battle over gender roles and women's self-determination is deeply ingrained in how we physically navigate the landscapes around us, and what those landscapes look like. In many places, our choices are constrained— without access to a car, we can become trapped in the home. But by using our limited resources on a car, we become trapped in increasingly deep poverty. Without access to reproductive choices, we are trapped with the de facto consequences of that lack of choice.

Meanwhile, the bicycle offers freedom. Damaged as our communities and bodies may be by the world that has been built around us, on a bicycle we can bridge the distances between physical places and break the limits we have set on ourselves. The bicycle is not for everyone, and it is not a solution in itself; but it is undeniably one of the most powerful tools we have available for our liberation.

Who is this book for? Everyone. Most books about bicycling happen to be written by, for, and about men, even if that isn't explicitly spelled out in the marketing materials, but that does not stop many women from reading them, and we aim to be no less inclusive. Most of our contributors identify as women, and the writing and art here describes our lives, our expertise, and the many things you too might experience or want to know about that you simply won't

find in other books or articles or even casual conversations about cycling. We aim to shift the tacit assumption that men are the experts, the audience, and the standard when it comes to cycling or anything else. And with that, we hope to help budge the idea that we must be defined by anyone else's ideas about what anybody's gender or our anatomy and reproductive capabilities mean.

We put together this book as a guide to some of the ways people use and think about bicycles as they relate to gender. We invited diverse perspectives and aimed to cover a lot of ground. Such a book could never be complete, and there are many gaps here that we hope you will be inspired to fill in with your own words and ideas. We hope that we have provided enough of an array that every reader will find something of practical use, something thought provoking and perhaps disturbing, and something to make you cheer.

We hope that you enjoy the ride.

A well-known riding teacher says that most of his women pupils take their first lessons in skirts on a woman's wheel. They go out on the road this way from three to ten times. They then come back to him in bloomers, learn to mount and dismount from a man's wheel, which is a great deal harder than the other way, and never again can be induced to ride a woman's wheel.

Girls who ride for pleasure like to ride with men, of course, and the only way to do it is to keep the pace they set. It cannot be done in skirts on a woman's wheel, and a man, even a polite escort, cannot be expected to ride slow forever, and so it happens that men's wheels grow more popular with women every day, and after awhile when people stop talking about it and the small boys stop hooting it will all be very charming and agreeable.

-San Francisco Chronicle, May 19, 1895

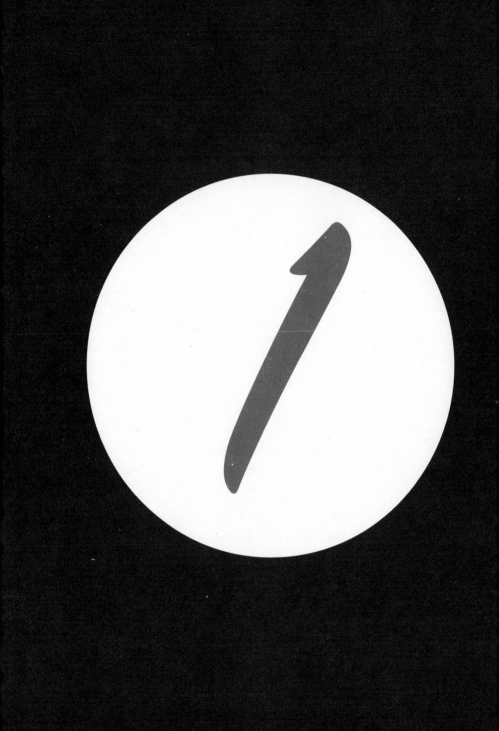

Knowledge

Is

Power

It's easy in any kind of conversation about gender—or any other sort of identity—to become overwhelmed by everything that is wrong: the microaggressions, the biases, the iniquities, the violence. As our eyes open and our brains wrap themselves around a new way of seeing that means judging things we used to take for granted. For a time, it's all we can see. Yet it's just as important to be able to see the other side of the coin: The forward thinking, the brilliantly disruptive, the visionary... and the opportunities around us to create something new, and to use what we know to make that new world better.

Critique is vital. And knowledge is power. But power also means being able to imagine a different world and to share that vision with others. If all we can see and share are the wrongs we're subject to, that can become as ultimately disempowering as not acknowledging them at all.

By all means, see what's wrong and say it loud. But don't forget to use that knowledge, however terrible, to give yourself a chance of something better, and to lead your community that way, too.

THE TRIPLE THREAT: SEXUAL PLEASURE, WOMEN, AND BIKE SEATS, FROM THE 1890S TO TODAY

Samantha Brennan

What do cycling and philosophy have in common?

It's a rather sad fact that two activities that make up a big part of my identity are heavily male dominated. It's not just a numbers thing. It's also that normative ideals of the cyclist and the philosopher are both gendered male in ways that make it hard for women to fit in and to count as philosophers and as cyclists. I'm interested in the historical connection between women, bicycles, and feminism—but my focus is really on the worry that women's bodies are unsuitable for riding, an attitude that formed part of the backlash to early feminism and one that I think carries forward today.

As the women's movement and the women's cycling movement gained traction, setting the New Woman on her course, there was considerable opposition to women's riding. Clearly, cycling was unladylike. There are many published speeches by clergy against the spectacle posed by women on bikes. Other clergy worried that access to transportation would make it easier for women to give into our baser natures and undertake morally loathsome activities, including prostitution and infidelity. I love the idea that women's sexuality is so wild and so corrupt that only lack of reliable transportation keeps us chaste and faithful. My favorite clergy quote, however, admits that cycling isn't always a bad thing: "The mere act of riding a bicycle is not in itself sinful and if it is the only means of reaching the church on a Sunday, it may be excusable." (1885)

Much more interesting from a philosophical point of view is the medical condemnation of women's cycling. Many physicians held that women's bodies simply weren't suited to cycling. The bicycle was a sure path to sexual depravity (given the motion of the bike and the proximity of the seat to women's genitals) and infertility (given the shaking the womb obviously endures while riding a bike). Also, our weaker natures made us prone to exhaustion. In "The hidden dangers of cycling," A. Shadwell, M.D, (1897) advised women against "attempting a novel and peculiar experiment with their precious persons." He wrote that the risks of cycling include internal inflammation, exhaustion, "bicycle face," appendicitis, dysentery, and nervous attacks.

One of the most striking things in the history of women's cycling is the terror of female masturbation associated with the shape and position of the bicycle seat. It's worse than the dreaded bicycle face, and worse than the fear that bicycling would make women prone to infidelity and prostitution.

Here's a passage from Peter Zheutlin's article, *Women on Wheels: The Bicycle and the Women's Movement of the 1890s*, that presents the general problem quite clearly:

"That bike riding might be sexually stimulating for women was also a real concern to many in the 1890s. It was thought that straddling a saddle combined with the motion required to propel a bicycle would lead to arousal. So-called 'hygienic' saddles began to appear, saddles with little or no padding where a woman's genitalia would ordinarily make contact with the seat. High stems and upright handlebars, as opposed to the more aggressively positioned 'drop' handlebars, also were thought to reduce the risk of female sexual stimulation by reducing the angle at which a woman would be forced to ride."

In "Reframing the Bicycle: Advertising-Supported Magazines and Scorching Women," Ellen Gruber Garvey (*American Quarterly*) writes that both critics and advocates of women's cycling used medical arguments related to women's sexuality and reproduction. Anti-bicyclists claimed that riding would ruin women's sexual health by promoting masturbation, while pro-bicyclers asserted that bicycling would strengthen women's bodies and make them more fit for motherhood.

Garvey is struck, like me, with the amount of ink that was spilt on this particular problem and the amount of detail regarding masturbation and evidence of masturbation that the doctors describe. It's not just the seat itself that's at issue. Doctors were also obsessively concerned with rider position. The same position that with men was associated with going fast and racing, was seen with women as an obvious aid to masturbation. Men who like going fast ride stooped over to dodge the wind, but when women adopted the same position, doctors assumed it was a means of getting more pressure on the clitoris from the bike seat.

So we can see two problems here with bike seats, the first is their shape and position, but the other concerns the posture of the rider. Sitting upright makes women go more slowly and is apparently less likely to provoke sexual excitement. Did anyone consider that the flushed face and the obvious excitement

of sitting in an aerodynamic racing position came from the thrill of speed? Probably not.

But surely the fear of bike orgasms has gone away? Right? Sort of. Every few years a version of the "women have orgasms while exercising" story goes around.

The triple threat of sexual pleasure, women, and bike seats is still a source of humor among cyclists. I was once on a ride where we encountered a section of road locals called "corduroy"—halfway paved, still bumpy. After we got to the end of it, one of the men at the front yelled back, "Do you girls want to ride over that section of road again?" Nervous laughter ensued.

The issue of contact with bike seats hasn't gone away altogether, either. Contrary to what most people think the best seat for fast riding is not a big, wide, comfy sofa of a thing. Instead it's a narrow, racing-style seat. Ideally for comfort you want as little contact as possible between your body's soft parts and the seat of a bicycle. The cut away styles of the 1800s are making a bit of a resurgence, and comfort, not fear of orgasm, is behind their sales. But sometimes I look at the cut out seats and think back to the 1890s and wonder if the doctors of the day would have smiled approvingly.

But of course it's better to fix the seat than surgically alter the rider. Cosmetic surgery wasn't an option in the 1890s but it is today. Cycling is frequently given as justification for labial trimming. And yes you read that right, cycling.

The Canadian Broadcasting Corporation's story on the increase in labiaplasty is typical. It begins with the story of a woman and her bike:

"Carrie Anne is a triathlete in her 40's, biking for 8 to 10 hours at a time but limited by the discomfort caused by the length of her labia. (Due to sensitivity issues and to protect her identity Carrie Anne is a fictitious name.) Thinking it was normal, she lived with it for years until finally getting a labiaplasty, a surgery that 'trims' the labia minora or inner labia, the external parts of the female genitalia."

"I was very uncomfortable," Carrie Anne said. She told CBC's *The Current* that the surgery is fantastic. "I just feel much more ...it sounds maybe weird to say, but attractive."

You might think that attitudes to women's bodies and cycling have changed in the serious cycling world. In reality, things are still grim. Extreme surgical intervention aside, it's regularly the case that women's races are shorter than those of the professional men. Women's bodies are sometimes still thought to be so delicate as to require shorter bike race and ride distances. A local event here, The Centurion, offered everyone the option of the metric or the imperial century, 100 km or 100 miles. But the event designated as the women's ride was only 25 km. It was also the only ride that was also a fundraiser for breast cancer research. The whole thing screamed pink.

We like to laugh at the anti-women's cycling backlash of the late 1800s—after all, bicycle face is a silly idea. But then why have we still not gotten over the idea that women's bodies aren't fit for bicycle riding?

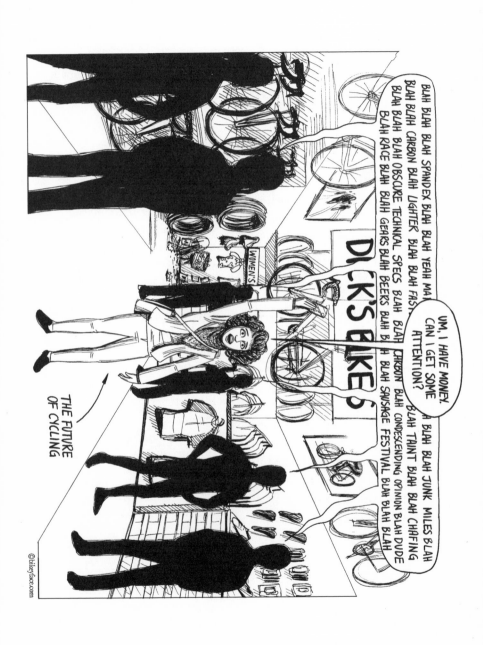

THE BIKE TEST

Elly Blue

This essay is based on a talk I gave at the first-ever Women's Bike Forum in September, 2012.

As the influence of women grows across all types of bicycling, so has the public debate about the representation of gender everywhere from ads to advocacy campaigns, race tracks to board meetings. Looking at a photo of a sexy woman on a bike, how are you to decide if is it sexist or empowering? Objectifying or compelling? Tokenizing or inclusive? Is it different if the photo was taken by a woman? What if the woman depicted is an avowed feminist? Does this mean we are never allowed to show women wearing skirts and heels? These discussions tend to get frustrating, in part, I think, because we don't always have a shared idea of what these terms mean.

I saw the need for an analytical tool that could be used by both media creators and consumers to evaluate images of women in bicycling. I was inspired by the Bechdel Test, which is named after a 1985 comic drawn by Alison Bechdel in her famous long-running *Dykes to Watch Out For* series, and attributed to her friend Liz Wallace. The comic shows two women coming out of a movie. "I have this rule, see," one is saying. "I only go to a movie if it satisfies three basic requirements. One: It has to have at least two women in it … who, two, talk to each other, about, three, something besides a man."

It's remarkable how many movies today still don't pass this simple test. Inspired by this metric, I came up with…

THE BIKE TEST.

Here are the criteria:

1. Are women present or represented at all?

2. Are the women presented as active subjects rather than passive objects?

3. If the gender were reversed, would the meaning stay more or less unchanged?

Going down this list is a surprisingly effective way to evaluate inclusiveness of a wide range of representations and entities, including advertisements, movies, news coverage, organizations, corporate or nonprofit boards, events, conference lineups, curricula...whatever happens to be in front of you. And needless to say, this all applies well beyond bicycling.

Here's a little more about each criterion, followed by examples. Some of the results may surprise you.

1. ARE WOMEN PRESENT OR REPRESENTED AT ALL?

I wish this didn't have to be on the list. Unfortunately, it still does.

I've been to panels of thought leaders and advocates where important ideas are being discussed—by men.

Shortly before I gave the presentation that this essay is based on, I read an (otherwise excellent and fascinating) interview with three luminaries in modern bicycle advocacy in the League of American Bicyclists' magazine, in which they reflect on the history of the bike transportation movement and how it got to be where it is today. It's full of dozens of names, and much of the purpose of the article seems to be these shout-outs, giving credit where it was due. Only one name, however, mentioned in passing, is female.

At the Women's Summit, someone waved a magazine in the air that had been left on one of the tables in the conference hall: A recently published road bike mag that contained not a single picture of a woman.

It's also interesting to note that most bike industry ads do not ever portray women unless they are for specific "women's" bikes and accessories... even if they aren't specifically for men either.

Of course the simple presence of a woman on stage, on the page, or otherwise in the limelight isn't a sign that an event is gender equal or gender neutral—in fact, arguing that it is often is the surest sign that it is not. But the sad truth is that in many cases even token representation is lacking.

So yes, we still do need this to be the first criterion. I look forward to the day when we can drop it from the list.

2. ARE THE WOMEN PRESENTED AS ACTIVE SUBJECTS RATHER THAN PASSIVE OBJECTS?

This one is trickier. One question to help hone in on this is: Are the women actually riding bikes, or just posing on (or near) them? Or better, is the woman the hero of her own story, or is she there to be drooled over?

It may help at this point to think this through using another excellent analytical tool, this one from the seventies: the Male Gaze. Coined by film theorist Laura Mulvey, the idea is that visual representations stem from and shape our identity, both as viewers and viewed. Mulvey points out that the view of the movie camera often represents the gendered assumptions of a heterosexual, white man. Movies then and now frequently portray women as passive objects with little agency or subjectivity of their own, often serving a similar function in the plot as, say, a pet, a statuette, a sled ... or a bicycle.

Advertisements fail this part of the test in droves. The landscape has improved since I wrote the original form of this essay, but eye-rolling moments still abound. Naked women. Naked women being grabbed. Naked women with miniature men riding across their bodies on tiny bicycles. Women in skimpy outfits, promising satisfaction. What do all these naked or nearly so women have to do with bikes? They're both objects that "you," the hetero/macho male audience presumed to be gazing upon them, might want to possess, I suppose.

Even ads that sell bicycles *to* women often flop here at step two; most are savvy enough not to sexualize their models, but rarely do they actually photograph the models riding the bikes. In the visual currency of the bicycle industry, men ride while women pose. Men act, women stand and watch. The reality of all too many races, meetings, and bicycling events is all too similar.

Another place this second part of the test fails with flying colors is in professional cycle racing. Take the Tour de France, in which only male athletes are allowed to compete—women are front and center during the award ceremony at the end as "podium girls," wearing cute branded miniskirts and kissing the race winners on the cheek as part of the spoils of victory. The role of the podium girls, in more or less skimpy attire, is an institution in the bicycle racing world, as is the equally demeaning job of "booth babe" at conventions and trade shows.

The male gaze can also be conveyed purely through text. The Cycle Chic website, which depicts fashionable women ("and men!" its proponents often chime in) riding bikes in cities around the world, does brisk business in merchandise that reads "Hold My Bicycle While I Kiss Your Girlfriend." Who is the presumed speaker here? Who is the presumed listener? Notice how the two objects of the phrase are interchangeable.

3. WOULD IT MEAN THE SAME THING TO THE SAME PEOPLE IF IT WERE ABOUT A MAN?

At the time I wrote this first blog post, a major bicycle manufacturer had taken out a two page spread in a magazine showing a woman in a hammed up "sexy nurse" costume bent over, pumping up the front tire of one of their new bikes. "Get sick soon," the caption urged.

This remains my favorite representation of the third part of the Bike Test. No huge amount of interpretation or skilled feminist analysis is needed to instantly recognize this as a demeaning and sexist ad. But it more or less passes the first two criteria: It shows a woman. And she's actively engaged in bike maintenance. If she were dressed like she was about to go tear up some sick singletrack, there would be nothing off about the ad. It's the decidedly non-medical miniskirt and low-cut top of the nurse's outfit that seals it. Imagine a man in her place, dressed up for Halloween. Imagine the discomfort—or horror, or perhaps just derision—of the same readers who are being invited to chuckle tolerantly and drool a bit at the image with the woman.

Promote an image that demeans men in the same way that it demeans women, and suddenly anyone can see it, and be indignant. Or replace a roomful of men with a roomful of women, as has been happening recently at some bicycle related events, and suddenly it's easy for everyone to see a gender disparity. That's the meat of this third point: If reversing gender roles makes a representation seem ridiculous, then it was already ridiculous—just maybe you hadn't noticed yet.

Of course, this is not all simply made and chosen by men. Women are also active in many representations of bicycling that would fail this test, as willing models, as photographers, as leaders and participants alike. My point is not that we are the helpless victims of sexist men, but that we're all part of a culture where sexism is normalized, celebrated, and rewarded.

It's also worth noting that while sexist representations actively sideline women, they don't really serve most men well, either. The macho culture promoted by much of the bike world (not to mention the rest of the world) is a burden to us all; we'd be better off without it.

There's a widespread sense that this is the game we have to play if we want to succeed. In a way that's true, but there are inherent limits for women in this game; we can only go so far. If we want something truly different, we need to change the rules.

If you're reading this, you're a consumer of media. You may very well be a producer of it as well, or at least a retweeter of it. It's up to all of us to do it better—let's start now.

I have a thing I do whenever I see other black people in places where there aren't a whole lot of us around. When possible, I make eye contact, give a nod and a smile, and sometimes I even say hi as I pass. Some people return the greeting, while others ignore me completely. I never know what reaction I'll get in return. I don't usually expect one—it's just one of the things I like to do as a way of saying "I see you, baby." I know I feel invisible when I'm out and about, so I do what I can to make sure I don't contribute to that feeling in others.

Earlier tonight while riding home, a black woman walked across the pedestrian crosswalk a few feet ahead of me. She was an immigrant like me, but from a different part of the world; I guessed Sudan as I got a good look at her. Black American immigrants have an easy tell; we swagger when we walk. This woman wasn't strutting. She was just making her way from one side of the street to the other the best way she knew how.

As I drew nearer, I nodded and smiled like I always do. She gave me a hesitant smile at first. Then a grin erupted across her face and a laugh escaped her lips. She saw the helmet, saw a black woman on a bike, and something about that, about me, filled her with such joy that she actually cheered and pumped her fist as I rolled past her. I couldn't contain my own enjoyment of her reaction, and as our laughter mixed on 10th Avenue, the ride up the hill seemed a little bit easier.

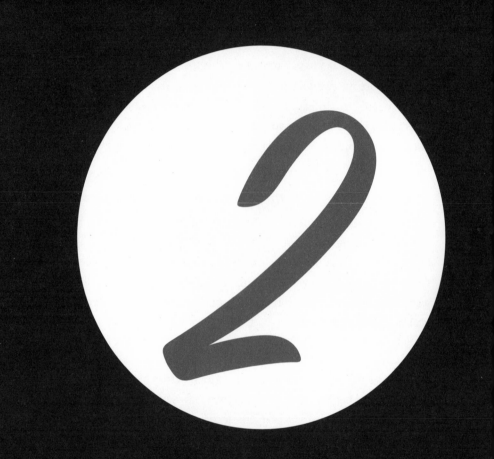

Being In Our Bodies

From a very young age, girls are conditioned to be ashamed of our bodies, to think of them through a critical, sexualized male gaze until we adopt that gaze as our own. Body consciousness is a factor that keeps many women off of bicycles. It doesn't help that many of the cyclists we see are squeezed into skin-tight uniforms. The advent of technical clothing for biking is welcome, though currently it isn't even manufactured in women's plus sizes.

If there's one thing we hope the women's cycling movement can do, it is to shift our culture so that it becomes very easy for anyone to get on a bicycle and ride strongly, without a second thought to what we look like to the people we pass by.

ON YOUR LEFT!

Adrian M. Lipscombe

When I showed up that morning, I knew what to expect. I knew this was going to be a long and tiresome journey; things would be confronted and said. I put on a face for you as harsh as the ride we are going to take. I needed to protect myself before this adventure.

Now you see me. I look nothing like you, and I never will. You see my bike. It is not like yours, and you judge me. Your eyes tell me that my bike and I don't belong. With one glance, you throw me in a cycle of no return. A cycle of loneliness and isolation; I knew I would be on this journey alone.

To you, I will be out of sight and out of your mind, even as I ride behind you.

If only you could see what I see, you might think differently.

You say this bike is not fit for me; I know you're wrong. You would never call me a cyclist of any kind; I know I am something you cannot define. I know, I just know, you think I am on my bike out of necessity.

From the beginning, bikes are specialized for you and not for me. I force my body to specialize instead, to conform and yield to the bike that was made for you. My bike cost as much as I weigh. My weight fights against the bike form as I demand this bike be tamed. Under me, my wild ride listens and creaks, calling out the pain and judgment we have received.

In my world, in my own time, you could see me for me. You will notice my skin goes for miles and is the color of my bike tires and as smooth as the grease on my chain. It grips my curves and calls out my differences to you. My veins pump the blood of my ancestors and my heart beats their drums. The sweat that beats down my skin perspires my oppression for being different. As it rains off me, it tastes of salt and sweet dreams, but stings my eyes with reality. It makes me glisten even at midnight.

As I draft behind you, I can feel the cold air riding between my fingers, asking me to let go. I grip harder to the handlebars that are leading my ride. I can feel the tape unraveling and my heart along with it.

My arms are long branches that are rooted from my shoulders

to the breasts on my chest. These arms hold me high. They bend to arch against this head wind, supporting my back that carries a weight I have been sentenced to my entire life.

I inhale deeply. We breathe the same air but I'm exhaling power. I fill my lungs with hope while pushing through to imprint my own tread in this world.

My thighs are thick and rub together with ease. As I pedal for miles, they swell and hug my frame protectively. I can flip the switch to provide propulsion to help me climb the hills of regret and doubt, and to pass anyone who doubts my power. These cages keep my feet in place but cannot cage me; they set me free.

I see my freedom ahead. My gears will grind and call out for mercy. I will shift speeds but never slow down to lose you. The triangulation of my pelvis has held life and it controls the world.

These wide hips are not made for this preformed saddle. I will wear down this hard cold leather to be soft and pliable to conform to me. As the miles mount, there is not enough padding in these shorts to protect me from the chafing of this ride. I will feel it for days after. It will pulsate from my

womb to my ass. I am a rough ride.

I look ahead and I see behind you. I see your fear of my wild, untamed mane wanting to be set free from this helmet. My hair unravels behind me, fighting with the wind to be free. Strains of my charcoal kinky curls sink down my face tracing the tributaries of sweat.

You're bewildered by my actions, by how I allow myself to be so free. This is not just a ride; this is a journey of empowerment. I break the circuit between us as I move to pass you, electricity lingering. Now we are side by side for a moment. For less than one second we are one, we are the same. We match speeds, breath, and we lock eyes. Now you see me and I see you. I open my mouth to feel the cold air rush between my pearls of wisdom and down into my lungs and I have the courage... the right... to say...

"On your left."

I look forward and see a clear path ahead, welcoming me to pedal forward to lead you. Before, I may have been on the same path as you, but now I know I am on a different journey. My journey is just beginning to change you and me. Allow me to blaze this trail for you.

Biking has freed me to see my body differently, at least most of the time. I used to look in the mirror and see the bulges on the outside of my thighs. Now as I pedal I look down and see strong, powerful legs. I could be self-conscious about the triceps that aren't as taut as they once were—but I know I can carry my fully loaded bike up a flight of stairs if need be, so I have strong, capable arms. I could worry about the size of my butt, or be glad I have some cushion for the saddle.

–Barb Chamberlain

MY BUTT

Nickey Robare

I never thought much about my butt before I started biking. I hated my boring straight brown hair, my big boobs, my jiggly belly, my eyes that would always need glasses. But I didn't hate my butt—it was neither great nor terrible, it was just the soft part of my body I sat on.

I always loved riding my bike. In high school I begged my mother to let me ride to school, but we lived in the city and my school was over five miles away, so she felt it was too dangerous. When I moved to Portland in my twenties I was free to do as I chose, and I started riding everywhere because the bus was too slow.

As I became regularly physically active for the first time in years, I discovered that my body was strong and could transport me almost everywhere I needed to go. My muscles grew strong and firm, and I began to love exercise. At times, I was still subject to dark thoughts about my body but I learned that the more I rode my bike, the less that happened.

I still didn't think about my butt much. A few years after I got into cycling I was discussing weight and size with a friend who had a very similar body type to myself. We both agreed that, overall, riding a bike for regular transportation won't really help you lose weight. "Honestly," she said "biking has just made my butt get *bigger*." I thought about it for a minute and realized, yeah, my butt had probably gotten bigger too.

A few years later, I moved away from Portland—a relatively flat city with a lot of long, gradual slopes—to hilly Seattle. It is *a lot* harder to be a regular cyclist in Seattle, but I did it, because I loved biking too much not to. To get to work I had to ride down one giant hill and up another. After a couple months of this I realized that I felt incredibly strong. One day I poked my butt and thought, *holy cow, that's solid muscle!*

I started noticing my butt more and more. Anytime I felt bad about my body I'd just look in the mirror and turn sideways to gaze at my butt. It was bigger than ever before, solid muscle, and just... fantastic. Once a friend got drunk and blurted out "Seriously, your butt is *out of control!*" When I went back to visit Portland I'd make my friends poke my butt so they, too, could marvel at its muscular force.

Despite my experience of sudden bootyliciousness, I would never suggest anyone start biking just so they can get a "nicer" butt. All our bodies are different, and there's no way to know if biking will make your booty bigger or smaller—although it's probably safe to say that it will make it stronger.

I didn't start biking with the hope that my body would change; I just needed to get around. In general, I think worrying about how you'd like your body to be different

is a useless exercise. Despite what we're constantly told by the media, permanent weight loss is nearly impossible. This is the body you've been given, and it's the only one you'll ever have. You might as well stop stressing about how you'd like it to be slimmer/taller/curvier/shorter/whatever and just learn to love it.

That's what cycling can do. There's no guarantee that it will change your body, but it can change your mind. It can teach you that you are stronger than you thought, and that even if you don't know how to love your body, it knows how to love you. It is capable of so much.

After a year in Seattle I moved back to Portland. I got an apartment one block from my office, so I biked a lot less. The muscles I had developed softened a bit, but I didn't really mind. I still enjoy my derriere—I had just needed a rock-hard push to start noticing it.

CYCLING UP AN APPETITE

Constance Winters

Some time ago in graduate school, a friend in the psychology department was conducting research on eating disorders. Her methodology called for interviewing female students with and without eating disorders, then comparing the two groups' narratives on several key topics. But when she set off to recruit participants for her study, she ran into a problem: of the several dozen young women recruited though a random selection process, all but one showed symptoms of disordered eating in the pre-screening interview!

She did not have a sufficient control group of healthy eaters. So she dismissed her initial participant pool and tried again, only to get a similar outcome. Eventually this led my friend to change the direction of her investigation. Her inability to recruit a group of university women with no history of eating disorders in itself became the theme of her research.

Looking back 10 years later, I am struck by another layer of irony in this story: I don't think my friend or I would have qualified for the study's control group ourselves. While neither anorexic nor bulimic, our eating was not what I would now consider normal. We were hyperaware of our calorie intake and we knew our precise weights. We paid attention to the times of day we ate and kept mental notes on the amount of exercise we'd need to do in compensation for every meal and snack. For non-nutritionists, we were far too well informed on the properties of various foods and their supposed effects on our blood-sugar and hormone levels. The truth is, eating at that age for many of us was an inherently conflicted experience, with food and its effects on our bodies lacing our inner lives with anxiety. We were not fashion models, movie stars, or athletes—we were university students. And for us it was not so much about our looks, as about grasping for control in a competitive and stressful environment.

I realize now, it was also a matter of having lost our natural appetite regulation mechanisms. We counted calories because we had gotten to the point where we genuinely could not tell when we were truly hungry and when we were not. Our hunger and satiation signals were so out of sync with reality that we no longer trusted them. At age twelve, feeling hungry simply meant I needed to eat something. But by the age of 22 this connection had been severed. Now there were nervous hunger, drunk eating, emotional eating, and comfort food binging. There were bread comas and sugar comas. There were the mid-morning shakes despite having eaten breakfast. Lack of appropriate satiation signals could lead to overeating unless we were vigilant, but being vigilant only perpetuated the cycle. And it all made us miserable.

How did this become the norm for so many women? Most likely it began with dieting in our teenage years and spiraled out from there, exacerbated by the sedentary lifestyle of the college student and office worker. We did not see ourselves as disordered because we were neither puking up food nor outright starving ourselves. We were simply "eating healthy," watching our weight. But in truth we were suffering and did not know how to put an end to it. In retrospect, I cannot believe how normalized this was in my generation. Countless male friends have told me that they've never had a girlfriend who was not "weird" about food.

It's hard to pinpoint exactly when things began to turn around for me. But it probably started with my move to a large, pedestrian-friendly city in my late 20s. Because of the city's layout and where my home and office were situated, I was suddenly doing lots of walking—not for the sake of fitness, but as a natural part of living and getting around. For the first time in my adult life, physical activity became integrated into my daily routines. It was no longer something I had to label "exercise" or "sport" and deliberately make time for. Over time, I found myself fixating on food less and enjoying it more.

It was riding a bicycle that truly accelerated the process of getting my appetite instincts back on track. When I first began cycling for transportation, it was a gentle, relatively short commute. Yet its physicality and the regularity of it was a shock to my system—and a welcome shock it was. In those first few months when I began commuting regularly by bike, I remember feeling as if my entire physical self was being ...*rebooted*, for lack of a better word. It was as if something that had been all but lost within me was now waking up, roused from a catatonic sleep.

Finding cycling enjoyable, I began to do it more—to rely on my bike entirely for getting around, and to go off on recreational jaunts in my spare time. It was then that I began to experience my body as a useful machine and not just a bothersome appendage to my brain. And it was then that I fully re-discovered food as fuel. If I wanted to ride, I had to eat.

It did not happen overnight. But little by little I found my hunger and satiation signals recalibrated, so that feeling hungry or full actually meant that I *was* those very things. I began to trust and appreciate my instincts. I began to trust and appreciate food. At the age of 30, for the first time in over a decade, I was able to eat when hungry and stop when full, just like I did as a child. Five years later, I am still happily pedaling and eating. I could not tell you how many calories a day I consume. I have not weighed myself in what must be a couple of years now. But I feel good, and the fact that my body and bike feel as one tells me I'm eating right.

OBESITY IS A BOGEYMAN

Heidi Guenin

I originally got into biking in Charlottesville, Virginia. I moved to an apartment that was on the edge of town if you looked at it from the perspective of a car window. Without a car, though, a small pedestrian bridge could cut miles off of the journey. I had been toying with the idea of giving up my trusty old Honda Accord, and I managed to snag a deal on a used electric bike that could haul me up the steep hill on the other side of the bridge.

Then one day, for reasons I can't remember now, I decided there was no reason I couldn't pedal up that hill under my own power. So I did.

My love of bicycling is part of what propelled me to pursue a career in public health. But somewhere along the way, I forgot that I started biking because it made me feel strong and powerful. I twisted around the cause and effect and started relying, at least professionally, on the idea that people should start bicycling to lose weight, to improve their bodies.

It's such a common argument that maybe you don't find it problematic. Ride a bike, lose weight, love your body. We all know people who can identify with that story arc. But the reality is that these people are the exception. Trying to get folks to ride a bike because they need to lose weight is scientifically and morally misguided.

Bicycling and other forms of physical activity are really good for you—no doubt about it, regardless of your weight. There's strong evidence showing that physical activity is positively associated with things like bone health and overall life expectancy, and negatively associated with heaps of poor health outcomes: Coronary heart disease risk, cardiovascular disease mortality, all-cause mortality, depression, hypertension, type 2 diabetes, osteoporosis, stroke risk, risk of breast cancer, colon cancer, and endometrial cancers.

In other words, hopping on a bike every day gives you a good chance of living longer and being happier and healthier while you're at it. Once we start considering the implications of reduced traffic crashes and better air quality, the case for getting to know your bike better is a damn strong one.

But what about obesity?

Obesity has become quite the public health bogeyman. Search for obesity-related popular media, and you'll get hit with "war," "crisis," and lamentations about how much it is costing our country.

Yes, there is plenty of literature linking obesity to various negative health outcomes, and this provides the foundation for most public health advocacy around physical activity. But a growing chorus of researchers is questioning the long-held and often-unwritten assumptions embedded in much of the existing obesity research—assumptions that can have devastating consequences for fat people.

One big assumption is the idea that being overweight is a health outcome in and of itself, meaning that losing weight is inherently good. Another is that physical activity will always lead to weight loss if you also eat well and have enough discipline.

These assumptions conveniently overlook the large number of metabolically healthy fat people. They ignore the different ways that different people's bodies handle fat. They create a foundation for fat-shaming, which is unfortunately still prevalent even in the medical establishment.

Shame and stigma are not effective tools for promoting health. And they're more than just ineffective—they're dangerous. And they don't work—low self-esteem is in fact associated with decreasing levels of physical activity. It doesn't take much imagination to understand why. Would you feel motivated to hop on a bike by a sense of not being good enough, prodded by the very folks who declared war against your body?

The research is skewed, as well. It simply doesn't occur to many researchers to include people in their studies who are both fat and healthy, which means that in studies that look at the benefits of weight loss, physical activity is often not controlled for. In fact, there is some evidence to show that being overweight or slightly obese is associated with lower mortality from all causes. That's right—it can be good for you to be fat.

Ultimately, I'm not suggesting that we ignore obesity altogether. But I am suggesting that we move

it way down the list. In our efforts to evangelize about bicycles and how much good they can do, obesity and its associated assumptions should never stand front and center—if they get mentioned at all.

Now I've returned to where I started. When I ride, I have fun, and I marvel at how far my body and my bike together can take me. Every once in a while, when I'm feeling particularly lazy and want to avoid riding, maybe I'll remind myself of the whole parade of health benefits. But I'm finished tarnishing my love of bicycling with the notion that it should be helping me lose weight. Now begins the much harder task of shifting the conversation within public health advocacy, where so many of these harmful messages have come from in the last decade.

BIKING THE TRANSITION

Nathan Ezekiel

I hit a rough patch when I was 18. I had recently come out as queer to my family—at the time, I identified as lesbian—and my parents were having a really hard time with it. Everything kind of snowballed. This was 1996, which now seems like a startlingly long time ago.

I dropped out of college and moved back to my hometown, Denver, Colorado. I got a job and was truly on my own for the first time in my life. There was no way I could afford a car, so I took the bus. Several months later, I was at my parents' house picking up some stuff and out in the garage I saw my childhood bike. It was a bright red Ross with 20" wheels and chrome fenders from about 1980. It had first belonged to my older sister, but all three kids in my family rode it at some point. It was still in good shape. I reclaimed it, fixed it up, and rode it all over town. Even that ridiculous tiny bike was faster than the bus.

The biking stuck. Biking was one of the few places I felt physically comfortable, like my body belonged to me. One aspect of my transness, which for me is a deeply physical thing, is that at least since puberty I've had a deep sense of alienation from my body—like it wasn't really mine. One of the ways I survived was by ignoring my body. I focused on other things—intellectual, artistic, and scientific things. Because my relationship with my body had always been like this, in some ways I didn't even notice it. All I knew was I loved how I felt on my bike, the feeling of doing something, getting somewhere. I loved the physical sensation of power and purpose.

My wife and I had always intended for me to carry our second child. Even though I couldn't pinpoint exactly what was broken, I thought the experience of pregnancy might be strong enough to fix my body. I thought that maybe if I could do this amazing thing that my body was built for, I might finally get it. I might feel like my body was mine. I'd always had problems with my cycle, and ovulated only rarely, so I went to acupuncture for over a year to get my body in shape for pregnancy. Between the indications I might have trouble getting pregnant and the extra pressure I was putting on myself to really get this right, I wanted to be as careful as possible. So when my acupuncturist told me I shouldn't bike while trying to get pregnant (or being pregnant), I listened to her.

I stayed off the bike for a year and a half. It was a brutal 18 months. My pregnancy would have been hard for anyone. I had health complications that were risky for our baby and the birth was hard, but it wasn't just that. Instead of the connection to my body that I'd hoped for, I felt deeper alienation. I had a lingering sense I was missing something important, that I wasn't supposed to feel this way. The kid was amazing, but I was miserable. I blamed it on not biking. I thought that if only I could have biked, maybe things would have been better.

Over time, my conscious awareness that I was male and that I needed to transition pushed to the surface. When I look back over my life "before," it's like most of it was in black and white. My senses, especially my physical senses, were muted and gray. But there were moments of color, moments where I felt alive and aligned. Many of those times happened on my bike. It wasn't until after I began to transition and realized what it could mean to truly live inside my body, that I understood there had been something strange about *only* feeling present in my body on my bike.

It's not so much that riding my bike was a part of my decision to transition. Rather, riding my bike was a glimpse into what my life could be. And to be clear, I'm not saying that I experienced (or now experience) biking as "male"—not at all. Instead, I'm saying that as someone who lived nearly my entire life completely separate from a sense of my body as my own, the time I spent on my bike was a respite. It was a feeling that I recognized as I transitioned and took up residence in my body again.

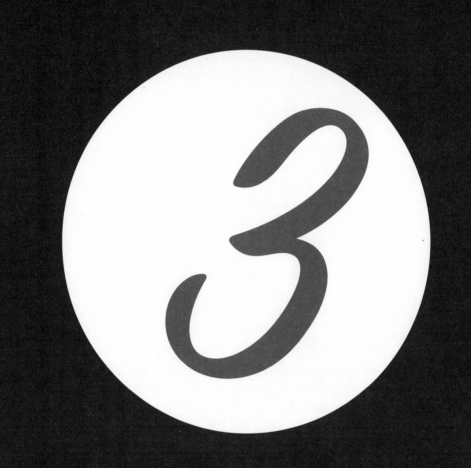

Safety

Whenever a conversation turns to women's cycling, the word "safety" always comes up eventually. But what does it mean? Not the same thing to everyone.

Often, it's about cars and the threat they pose to our vulnerable bodies on the roadway. Underlying this there's a debate about whether or not there is a gender gap in fear... are women more risk averse, men more foolhardy? Or, as we've been told not-quite-in-jest, are women simply smarter? Or is it that because we are more likely to carry (or at least be the primary caregivers for) children, we are the ones with the most to lose? Or perhaps, as some studies have suggested, women are more willing to admit to fear, so we get all the credit for having it.

Other times, when we talk safety we're talking about a more overtly gendered safety, and the threats of catcalls, street harassment and worse that women face all too often when we venture out into public spaces.

Ultimately individuals have their own thresholds for what feels safe. Often it's the small things that sway our decisions about how and when and where to move about in the world, rather than bigger-picture trends or fears. The contributors in this section offer some less-gendered but no-less-relevant ideas about feeling safe, comfortable, and secure on your bike.

THE AHA MOMENT

Echo Rivera

I enjoy the smooth riding that road bikes can provide, but sometimes I just want to speed through the woods and get dirty. A recent gorgeous day outside demanded that we do just that. We chose a trail that, according to the *New York Times*, is a "pretty nice mountain biking trail."

We entered the trail and, much to my delight, rode up on a small family of deer chomping down on some grass. Off to a great start!

We pedaled on through woods and smiled at wildlife—deer, squirrels, rabbits. I could hear birds and the slow churn of our wheels on the dirt. It was hard to believe that such an oasis existed close to the city.

Soon we approached a gravel hill that takes you over the highway. Jason sped ahead, as if it was no trouble. I, on the other hand, felt like I was trying to ride in quicksand. My heart was pounding so hard I thought it was going to explode.

"What's your problem?" I thought to myself. "It's just a stupid hill! You've done hills a hundred times!"

Yet, the crunch of the gravel stabbed at my mind. An agonizing cruunch-cruuuuncchh-cruuuuncchhhh, as sweat dripped off my forehead. My muscles were frozen in place. By the time I coasted downhill, I was irritated and had to fight a small urge to lunge my bike into Jason's just to end the ride. Instead, we crossed the road at the bottom of the hill and kept going.

I didn't like that stretch. It was dark. I could both see and hear the traffic. It was muddy and I almost fell thanks to a rock. And I was annoyed. At what, I didn't know, but I was annoyed just the same.

We came to the next stop, which requires one to either cross the road or go under a bridge. The bridge was muddy and flooded.

I stomped and grunted, "I don't like this side."

"We can go back if..."

"*Yes.* Yes I want to go back, let's go."

I was already turning around before he could say anything else. I was glad to be heading to the other side...and yet, I was really dreading that hill.

As I approached the top of the hill for the second time, something clicked in my head. It was so sudden that it was almost audible.

It's the gravel. It was the sound of wheels on gravel that upset me.

My car crash.

Just over ten years ago, exactly two weeks after getting my drivers license, I was in *(read: caused)* a head-on collision. I was trying to turn left, darted out too far forward, turned, and my tires spun out in gravel. I didn't know what to do, and whatever it was I did to react shot me into the oncoming lane. It was a nasty crash and I almost lost a leg (not to mention my life). Luckily, no one else was seriously injured.

The crash had a major impact on me. I could still drive, but I had nightmares and was easily startled. Driving by a crash would bring me to tears and put me in a solemn mood that could last for hours. I allowed only a select few people to drive me anywhere, and rewarded them with my nervous, jumpy, "*watch out!*" attitude and shrieks. Over time, these symptoms faded, except for the aching knee. But every now and then, something breaks through the old mental wounds and shakes me right up.

Like the sound of gravel on that hill, on that trail, on that day.

Once I realized what was wrong, my fear evaporated. I grabbed my handlebars and charged over that hill. It was as though I was pedaling through all the pain caused by that stupid, long-ago crash. It felt like if I pedaled fast enough, the painful memories would be left behind in the dust.

At the bottom of the hill, relief rippled through me, making the hair on the back of my neck stand up. I smiled and continued pedaling. We passed wildlife and people walking on the path as we pedaled our way back home. Everything the same. No one noticed that I just battled an internal evil—and won!.

At the last turn before reaching the road, I was treated with a watchful but trusting deer who allowed me to snap a picture.

I've thought about this day a lot—about how all sorts of things can be triggers or reminders of a traumatic event. For me, on that day, the sound of the gravel served as the conduit for my memories to come flooding back. But I have also thought about how I conquered the hill, gravel and all. I did not let it consume me. Riding my bike got me through it.

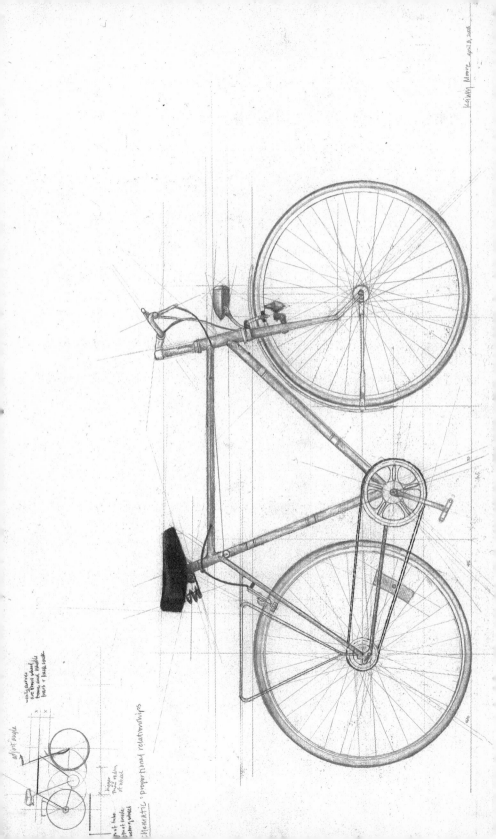

EVERYTHING YOU WANT TO KNOW ABOUT BIKING SAFELY

Alex Baca and Bec Rindler

BEC: Alex, hello! We write a series of conversations for The Billfold (.com) about biking and money. When we asked readers for questions, they focused on comfort and safety. These topics are all related because attending to comfort helps people feel safer and ride their bikes more.

ALEX: I truly believe that the number one way to be safe on a bike is to ride a bike that fits you and that you're comfortable on; that means having a properly adjusted seat, seatpost, and handlebars, but I can also talk about the importance of and variation in frame geometry and wheel size for days. I am hardcore about bike fit—and really, a professional bike fit is best, though those don't come cheap. If your bike doesn't fit right, you'll be fidgeting and thinking about how your back hurts or about how you're reaching too far with your legs or arms—and you'll be less inclined to pay attention to what's going on around you. Like traffic. And other cyclists. And traffic lights, and signs, and whatnot.

BEC: Yes, your senses are your best safety mechanism. I recommend buying things that heighten your ability to use them, like lights, and staying away from things that don't, like wearing earbuds in both your ears!

ALEX: As far as things I've bought for safety, I have a set of four LED, USB-rechargeable lights, which are stupid-easy to take on and off (leave 'em on and they might get stolen). I also put on really solid tires to avoid frequent flats.

BEC: Unsurprisingly, because we're friends who enjoy talking about biking, we have a lot of the same stuff! We both use Bern helmets to protect our noggins. I also use Gatorskin flat-resistant tires, and that helps me feel safer that I won't get stranded somewhere when I'm biking in unknown areas. I have a Knog Blinder for the front of my bike and a silicone blinky light for my seatpost. And I'm not sure you'd be caught dead wearing this, but I bought a neon safety vest that makes me feel more confident riding at night.

Let's give the readers some of our favorite tips about safety! We've mentioned things like lights and wearing neon (or at least light colors) that can help with night biking. I think knowing your route goes a long way towards keeping you safe. Practice, practice, practice—and get a buddy. I had a friend show me his commute when I first moved to New York, and I rode with a group of bikers who commute together who I found through the Bikeapolis website— these were my training wheels for biking by myself in the city. The other bikers recommended routes and told me about pitfalls (dangerous patches, ticketing cops), which helped me get more comfortable and feel safer. If you are thinking about bike commuting to work, I advise trying out your route on a weekend or non-rush hour time as a trial run. Start small. Bike to a friend's house. Then bike one way to work and take the bus home. The next day, do the reverse. Don't give up if you can only do it one or two days a week. That's a great start!

ALEX: My former coworker has been writing some smart blog posts about simple tips to make biking easier and more fun as part of the Washington, DC-based Women & Bicycles program. I recommend checking those out and keeping in mind that it's paramount to ride something that's safe and comfortable for you. Better tires, a nice bike seat, and bright lights might cost you more money than their lower-end counterparts, but they're worth it if you're riding longer distances or in the dark. (Talk to me about my Lumina 650!) Keep in mind the basic bike check: air, brakes, cranks, and chain. I have a personal checklist of things I think about before I get on my bike: Do my tires have air? Do I have a light (on my bike or on my person to put on my bike)? If I'm riding a significant distance, do I have what I need (15mm wrench, travel pump, tire lever, spare tube, multitool) to fix a flat or fix my bike if something goes wrong? Do I know where I'm going and do I have a cue sheet if I need one?

Once I get on my bike, I make sure that my brakes are working, that my seat is properly adjusted, and— because I ride a single-speed— my chain is tight. If anything feels weird, I fix it! I will say that a helmet is the absolute last thing on my personal safety checklist because I want to ensure that I've done literally everything possible to *prevent* an accident. Strapping on a foam bucket, however powerful it may be in the event of one, *will not prevent an accident.* I suspect many riders think they're totally fine because they've got a helmet on and overlook other really important things that could keep them safe—and alive. Make sure your accident-prevention game is on lock—with a comfortable bike, lights, properly inflated tires, and a solid sense of direction—before you put on a helmet. And make sure that helmet fits properly. Use the two-finger test.

BEC: One aside: Someone asked about biking home from the bar and, in general, alcohol consumption when you're biking. While a low-alcohol cocktail like a white wine spritzer might seem appropriate, it's a good idea to familiarize yourself with the alcohol laws—and all laws—in your area.

ALEX: Your local bike-advocacy group likely has a comprehensive list of laws for your jurisdiction. If you've

got specific questions about safety as it relates to local laws or procedures, contact them! Bike advocates are friendly people and are trained to answer your questions (though we typically can't dispense legal advice)! Most local organizations, especially in denser, urban-er areas, are focusing heavily on biking for transportation rather than, like, getting roads closed on the weekends for Cat 2 racers. This is, I think, a good thing.

Don't want to ride in traffic? Take the lane. *Take the goddamn lane!* It's scary at first, because cars will probably honk at you, but if you're worried about a car not seeing you, intentionally buzzing or grazing you, or forcing you to the right on a street with no shoulder, the absolute best thing you can do is get in the middle of the travel lane and ride at a steady speed. It's legal, and likely the worst that can happen is you'll piss off someone who was probably looking for an excuse to honk their horn anyway.

BEC: And we could write a whole piece about people we've pissed off in traffic, but let's just close with: You can do it! You can be comfortable and safe, and look good, and do it all on a bike for not too much money.

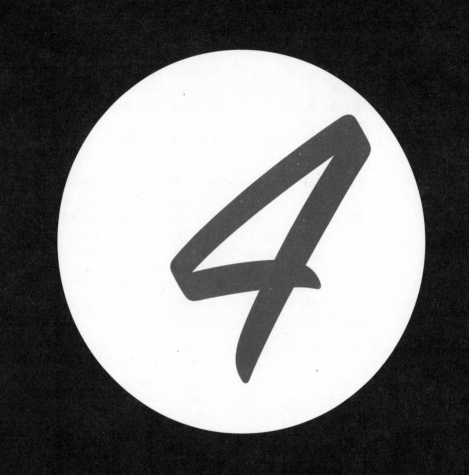

Clothes

*W*hat to wear is a dilemma that cycling often poses. "Just wear anything!" has always been our rallying cry, but that doesn't work for every person or every situation. Professional women, already facing the uncomfortable reality that we're earning less than our male colleagues, must manage a double standard for appearance and comportment to get and subsequently hang onto embattled jobs. In that light, questions of sweat, mascara, and hairstyles don't seem so trivial. Fortunately, many a stalwart pioneer in heels and a suit have paved the way and are willing to share their hard-won advice.

PEDALING AND PROFESSIONAL ATTIRE: NOT JUST FOR MARY POPPINS!

Constance Winters

As a professional woman who, for the past five-and-a-half years, has relied solely on her bicycle for getting around, I am no stranger to pedaling in a skirt-suit. And why not? Utility cycling is a means of transportation, not a sport. Most of us would not wear jogging clothes to walk to work, and neither would we don a special motoring costume to drive there. So why would I change just to cycle to a meeting? So yes: skirts, dresses, heels, overcoats—I wear it all, preferring to cycle in my everyday clothing to having to change at my destination.

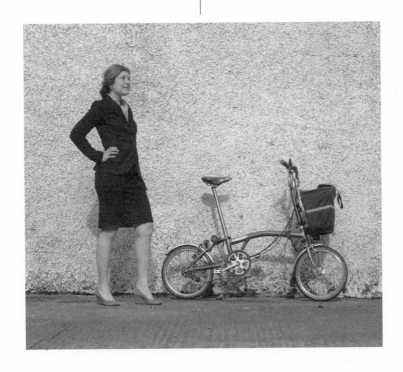

Admittedly, when it comes to "everyday clothing," professional attire is at the extreme end of the spectrum and presents its own set of challenges. The way I see it, these fall into two general categories, the first being comfort on the bike. "Isn't cycling in a suit awkward?" is a question I am commonly asked. Well, that depends on the suit. True, the combination of fabrics and tailoring used in professional attire often restricts your reach and pedaling motions, which is uncomfortable as well as unsafe. But not all clothing is made in the same way. The trick is to weed out styles that prevent a full range of movements. I will go through some basic wardrobe pieces to provide examples:

TOPS

When it comes to blouses, blazers, and coats, opt for those that do not pull at the shoulder seams when you extend your arms to grip the handlebars. The easiest way to ensure this is to look for garments with stretch in the fabric. However, even garments with no stretch can be tailored in such a way as to offer give in the shoulders. When considering a top, try it on, extend your arms as you would when gripping the handlebars, and see how it feels. Remember, the more leaned-over your cycling position is (for example, if you're riding a bike with drop bars), the more give you will need here.

SKIRTS

Overall, I find that skirts are surprisingly comfortable to cycle in—as long as you avoid styles that restrict pedaling. The infamous pencil skirt (a figure-hugging, extremely narrow style that hits at or below the knee) is the most obvious offender. The rule of thumb is: Choose a skirt that will allow you to open your legs! The classic A-line works best; luckily this is one of the styles most common to suiting. Pleated skirts, as well as skirts with slits at the back or sides, work well too.

A side note here: A bicycle with a step-through frame will dramatically expand your skirt selection, as it eliminates the need to swing your leg over the back.

TROUSERS

If you can wear ordinary slacks and jeans on the bike, there is really nothing unique about the more formal variant. One thing to watch out for, though, is a wide trouser cuff: Unless your bicycle is equipped with a chaincase or chain guard, a wide cuff can get dirtied—or sucked in!—by the chain. Avoid the wide-legged style, or else tighten your right cuff using a safety pin or a strap.

SHOES

For those who have not done it before, cycling in high heels might seem intimidating, but I would venture to say this is largely psychological. Assuming that you can cycle in flat shoes, there is absolutely nothing about a high-heeled shoe that is different, since it is the ball of your foot, not the

heel or the arch, that contacts the pedal—and this part of a shoe is no different for heels than it is for flats. Another issue is that dressy shoes—regardless of heel height—tend to be slippery. But if you are willing to spend $10, there is an easy fix: Take your shoes to a cobbler and ask for non-slip soles. Problem solved.

So, now you've got your cycling-ready professional wardrobe in order. But will it still look presentable by the time you arrive at your place of work? This is something that many novice cyclists ask about. I will break it down into specific points of concern.

WRINKLAGE

How do you wear nice clothes on a bike without looking wrinkled and disheveled? There are several aspects to achieving this. First, when cycling for transportation you need not ride with the same vigor as you would on a club ride. Think of cycling to work as the two-wheeled equivalent of *walking*, not running. You should be able to do it without destroying your outfit. A comfortable, upright bicycle with a wide saddle will also help keep you wrinkle-free, as your position will resemble sitting on a chair. Finally, you will find that certain fabrics (such as wool and cotton jersey) resist wrinkling, whereas others (such as crinkled linen) "feature" wrinkles as an inherent part of their design. As with everything, a bit of trial and error is needed, but over time you will develop an intuitive way of determining whether a garment will withstand your two-wheel commute.

SWEAT STAINS

Even when you take it easy on a bike, sweating is often unavoidable. But early on in my commuting adventures I discovered an easy fix: Wear prints. Yes, this really and truly works to disguise sweat stains! The best types of prints are fine and detailed with some tonal variation. Florals, paisleys, fine plaids, and intricate geometrical patterns are all good candidates. Stripes and polka dots can work as well, but in general the busier the print the better, tricking the eye into not noticing the tonal variations from sweat stains. It may seem too simple of a solution, but it is ridiculously effective: You can walk into a meeting straight off the bike wearing a sweat-soaked blouse and no one will be the wiser.

BODY ODOR

If you haven't discovered this already, avoiding synthetic fabrics—polyester and acrylic in particular—will curb BO to a degree that will surprise you. And, at the other end of the spectrum, wool is a fabric that almost magically resists odors. More and more wool active wear manufacturers are now making attire suitable for a professional setting, from button-down shirts to dresses.

STAYING DRY IN WET WEATHER

To keep your top half dry in the rain, look for a lightweight raincoat that is roomy enough to fit over a blazer. You can keep your hair dry with a hood or hat (I find classic wool berets to be amazingly water resistant—I tuck my long hair into mine and it stays dry for commutes of up to two hours). And the combination of nylon stockings and a skirt will keep your bottom half much dryer than trousers.

KEEPING HAIR PRESENTABLE

Over the years I've cycled for transportation, I've tried both long and short hairstyles. Personally, I find my hair easiest to manage when it is long: I simply tie it up in a bun and it's a fairly low maintenance transition from bike to office. If you wear a helmet, go for a low bun that can sit beneath it. And, if you can pull it off, many long-tressed cyclists swear by "Heidi braids" for a stay-put, muss-resistant look. Shorter hair can be kept in place with pins and berets. Ultimately, hairstyles are too personal of a thing to offer meaningful advice on, but if you approach cycling to work as transport rather than sport, you may find that keeping your hair presentable is not as daunting as you might have imagined.

More than anything, I find that the key to dressing professionally on the bike is in our attitude toward cycling. In cultures where cycling is predominantly viewed as a sport, the sight of a woman pedaling in a skirt and heels is unusual and has been known to evoke shouts of, "There goes Mary Poppins!" But it need not be that way, and the more of us who do it, the less unusual it will become. If you wear professional attire to work, you can still get there on two wheels—and feel all the better for it!

DRESS FOR SUCCESS ON THE BIKE

Janet LaFleur

Four years ago I made a commitment to ride my bike to work every day in my work clothes. I had seen photos and read stories of women in cities like Chicago and Boston riding dressed for work on cold, snowy days and hot, rainy ones and thought, *"What's my excuse here in California, where it's cool in the morning and doesn't rain all summer?"*

On that first day I put on a dress, a typical choice for my job as marketing director for a small software company in Silicon Valley, and hopped on an old mountain bike that I had souped up with a rear rack, boxy grocery panniers, and cheap flat pedals. With a cardigan on top for the morning chill, bike shorts underneath for modesty, and my laptop in one pannier and heels in the other, I effortlessly pedaled the five miles to my office on neighborhood streets. It only took 10 minutes longer than if I had driven.

Sweat was the enemy and I learned quickly how to avoid it. I'd pedal slowly, and if I started feeling the slightest bit warm I'd pull over, remove a layer and toss it in my pannier. When I arrived at work, I'd take a moment outside to remove my helmet, toss my hair, change into my heels, and cool down before I pushed my bike into the building.

Over time, I refined my tactics. I added a front basket so I could stash my sweater or scarf without stopping. I ditched the clunky grocery pannier for a more professional, bike-specific briefcase. I walked out without my flats one day and learned I could ride in high heels. I bought a trench coat for rainy days and a long wool coat for the winter. I fell in love with a cherry-red upright Dutch bike that made me feel elegant and dignified as I pedaled it on the test ride. I felt frivolous buying it, but it came with tangible benefits. Not bending forward meant my dress didn't hike up as much. And it had a chain guard, so I didn't have to tie back my dress pants anymore to keep the fabric out of my chain.

I didn't fully appreciate the power of a pretty bike until my company went through a shakeup. Tall, distinguished-looking board members roamed the hallways and hot sports cars and luxury sedans were parked out front. A new CEO was hired, then rumors of a buyout rumbled about. Appearances mattered, so I took extra care with what I wore and I was grateful to be riding an eye-catching, classy bike. Much as executives in the tech industry might talk about green programs, and as much as hoodies and jeans may be the norm for programmers, arriving at work on a beater bike wasn't going to raise my profile as marketing professional, regardless of what I was wearing.

The new CEO and visitors were intrigued by my Dutch bike: *"Where did you get it?" "Is the leather saddle comfortable?" "How many gears are in the internal hub?"* And the inevitable, *"You didn't actually ride in that dress and heels, did you?"* Commuting by bike went from a potential career liability to an asset as a conversation starter.

Buying a fancy bike isn't that expensive either when you compare it to buying a car. The cost of upgrading your SUV to leather seats would pay for a fully-loaded city bike. The extra cost of buying a BMW instead of a Camry would pay for a high-end road bike. And if you share a car with a significant other instead of buying a second car, you could afford all three: an upgrade to a luxury car, the road bike and the city bike.

In the end the company was sold, the marketing group was eliminated, and the CEO and board members moved on to other ventures. But when I searched for a new job, I had made all these new connections to tap into for job leads. And I had the confidence to ride my bike to the first day on the job at my new company.

EVERY SEASON

Elly Blue

SPRING

Climb into your jeans, the ones with the thrice-mended crotch, roll up your right pant leg, or both legs if you value symmetry, and pedal off down the road through the spectacular spectrum of cherry blossoms, sneezing.

Stop when you see a tell-tale cardboard box on the grassy strip in front of an apartment building. Rummage through the ugly vases, water-stained VHS tapes, and broken wicker baskets. Pull out the faded black scoop-neck shirt from beneath the rest of the crap and investigate it. If it only needs a wash and a little mending, shove it to the bottom of your pannier and keep riding.

SUMMER

Pull on the free box shirt, which you have not mended, over the flowered skirt that doesn't go with it but has gloriously capacious pockets. Slip into your flip-flops and pedal off down the road, not forgetting your keys, wallet, chapstick, and water. Feel electrified by the heat. Bring a thick sweater and leggings to prevent your body from getting accustomed to the air conditioning at work.

Summer is hard on clothes. It's a race to wear less of them and to sweat more in what remains as you pedal furiously downhill to the river and jump in. Wear the scuffs and tears and faded bits proudly, badges of your honorable wasting of your prolonged youth, your lack of ambition, your inability to sit at the table long enough to want to flip it over.

FALL

It's beginning to get brisk out, so ride as fast as you can everywhere you go, arriving sweaty and glowing with triumph. Graciously, breathlessly accept the attentions of the doe-eyed admirers who gravitate towards you in these moments.

Your coworker informs you that you need a technical rain jacket with a long butt flap, rain pants, fenders for your bike. As they speak, you observe the distant look in their eye, like they're reading from a teleprompter. Wear a cotton sweater and jeans every time it rains until even you have to admit discomfort, at which point spend a grudging $25 on a poncho and a pair of rubber boots at the army surplus store.

WINTER

You own a parka but you swelter in it any time you do anything more active than standing at a bus stop. One day, suddenly overpowered by the smell of stale sweat, leave it on the bus bench and walk away, free and unencumbered. The next morning, put on every sweater, sweatshirt, and pair of leggings you own and set off by bike. When you arrive at work, your layers of discarded clothing take up a footprint on the floor the size of a small natural disaster.

All winter, the wind tries to creep through every opening in your clothing, the gap between your sweater and jeans, between the seams of your gloves. Stay a step ahead of it, adding layers until you look like a multi-colored traveling circus. There's no way you can stay warm, even so. Instead, keep moving, riding late into the night to investigate the contents of grocery store dumpsters, beer bottles, and new acquaintances' basement bedrooms.

SPRING

As the weather warms up, shed your layers. By now they have become ragged, so instead of stashing them in a drawer in your tiny studio apartment, abandon them in the free boxes that are starting to appear again along your routes, different boxes than the ones you gleaned them from in the first place, thus completing the natural cycle of life, the turning of the seasons.

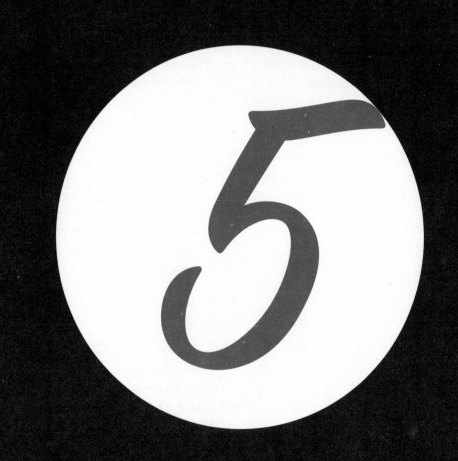

Vulva

Where the body meets the bike seat: If there were ever a taboo topic, this is it. Now we are getting beyond gender differences and into the stuff of biology. And yes, it's different for vulvas. Read and learn!

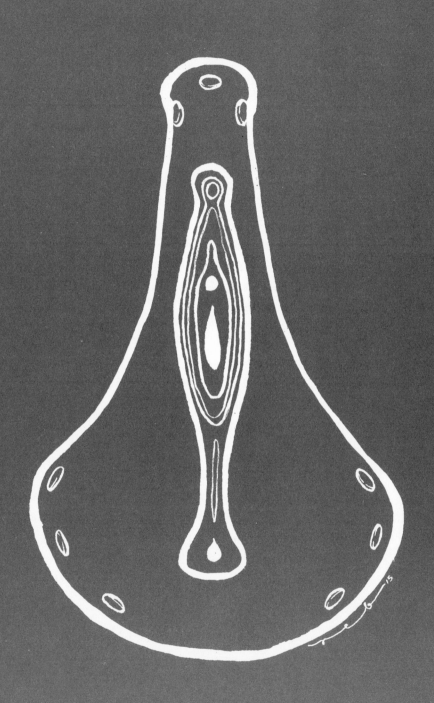

HOW TO MAKE YOUR BUTT HAPPY (ON AND OFF THE BIKE)

April Streeter

The word for heart in Swedish (*hjärta*) is close in both spelling and pronunciation to the word for ass or butt (*stjärt*). Perhaps this is one reason that classic Swedish outhouses have a carved heart on the door. Upside down, of course, this symbol of love looks remarkably butt-like.

The linguistic heart-butt connection may be why Swedes seem handy with bike saddle covers, especially butt-warming soft furry covers (yes, it's cold in Sweden).

Sweden is where I learned to love bike riding. After a not-too-happy initiation into road riding in my 20's, I had pretty much rejected cycling. Then, happily, I married a Swede who didn't think bike riding was something you necessarily needed Lycra or superhuman endurance to do.

Everybody bikes in Sweden and so I biked, too—and was happier for it.

Yet not even the Swedes seem to fully grasp the importance of a well-fitted saddle to your butt's—any butt's—ultimate bike happiness.

The reason the happy-butt issue is so neglected is a combination of confusion and (of course) cash. Many bicycle saddles are designed by and for men, and with disregard for all the different sore spots—from butt to labia to clit—that women can experience from a poorly fit saddle.

Strangely though, while the outer appearance of women's and men's genitalia is obviously different, internally the shape of the pelvic girdle and the distance between the sit bones, which determines what saddle length and width will be most comfy, is remarkably gender-neutral. Men may, in very general terms, have more narrow pelvic structures and women more generous ones, but men can also have wide ones and women narrow ones. It is your ischial tuberosities (and even more specifically the ischial rami) and the distance between them that partially determines how saddles will feel. You definitely want a saddle wide enough to accommodate these sitting bones.

Your bike and your style of riding also help determine how your butt feels after many miles of pedaling. For example, on road bikes you'll be leaning further forward than you would on a bike made for city cycling, so the touch point of your pelvis to the saddle will be moved—it could actually be your pubic symphysis that is touching down.

In short, there is a perfect saddle for every butt, but no one saddle will be perfect for all butts. Thus the best rule in having a happy butt is to get yourself a bike fitting. A bike fitting helps you make all the minute adjustments to your bike, such as how far up or down and also forward or back a saddle should be situated for your body.

After you have that perfect fit of your entire body to your bike, then you can work on a happy butt.

If it's possible, find a woman-supportive bike shop that has a saddle library. A saddle library is a collection of bike saddles that you can check out and try on your own bike, for a little fee. While Gladys Bikes in Portland, Oregon wasn't the originator of the saddle library concept, they offer one of the best. For $25 (applicable to your final purchase) you can take different saddles out for a few days each and really give them a good try before you determine what you want to buy.

As a cyclist and a yoga teacher, I think about the sitting bones quite a lot—and talk about them. At almost every yoga class, I can be heard telling people to 'feel your sitz bones' or 'pull the flesh from the sides of the thighs to feel your sitz bones more firmly connect to the ground.'

You could almost say I used to be smug about sitz bones. I had my well-broken-in Brooks saddle, and so most of the time my butt was pretty happy.

The Fates and the Furies, of course, do not like that kind of hubris. Pride goeth before a fall, or in this case, pride goeth before a sore butt. Because...I bought a new bike. A very cool, new-to-me electric cargo bike with 8 speeds and a powerful throttle for zooming me up hills with yoga mats and accoutrements on board.

Yet instead of heeding all that good advice I detailed above, I just rode this new/old bike with the squishy, worn-down-by-someone-else's-butt saddle from the previous owner. I successfully ignored the pain in the butt

this saddle was causing me. I would squirm around as I rode, trying to keep my soft tissues comfortable.

The discomfort did not go away and my pleasure at riding my new bike dimmed. I was able to semi-ignore the issue for many, many months. Until one drizzly winter day I came out of yoga class and loaded my mats into the front bike bucket. I unlocked the bike and wheeled it out onto the asphalt. Swinging a leg over the frame, my foot met pedal and I pushed off, sat down, and...squish. My butt, sans any rain pants, sank into the cold, wet surface of the padded saddle. My soft tissues were instantly painfully soggy and remained that way for some time that day.

It was a small misery to be sure, an insignificant misery in the greater arc of life, but big enough on that wet day to spur me finally to action. I went to the saddle library, looked over the choices, sat on some saddles, and made my decision.

And while I'm still in the breaking-in period for my new (different model) Brooks saddle, soft tissue squishing is a thing of the past. Happy butt is here again, both on and off the bike.

YOUR VULVA

Elly Blue and Caroline Paquette, RN retired, BSN

Still shadowed by man's heavy thumbprint on cycling, women have yet to enjoy decades of gender-specific research, or even coalesce and proudly announce our range of gender-specific on-the-bike needs. Never mind how men get comfortable in the saddle. How do women get comfortable?

We are excited to join a surge of interest in female-specific cycling product and knowledge. So we have joined up to offer a roundup of advice for bicyclists with vulvas, drawing from personal experience, conversations with friends, medical training, and the Internet. Hold onto your seats!

First, a quick anatomy lesson. Put simply, the vulva is the flesh around the entrance to the vagina. It includes the mons pubis (often called *mons veneris* or "Mound of Venus" for ladies; it's the padding over the pubic symphysis), the clitoris, and two sets of labia (that's Latin for "lips"). The outer set of lips are the *labia majora*, hair-covered fatty skin folds which derive from the same embryonic tissue as the male scrotum. The inner set, the *labia minora*, are thin, delicate, hair-free skin folds. The *labia majora* and *minora* come in an incredibly wide variety of color, fattiness, hairiness, and length, all of which are normal.

The entire vulva is prone to pressure, friction, and chafing while bicycling. Chafing can cause swelling, ingrown hairs, and sores—all sad, but very solvable. If you're in pain, experiment with your options. Start by reading this through, then by broaching the topic with other women who ride. There's a lot of knowledge hidden away out there, as well as a lot of unnecessary labial discomfort being awkwardly concealed. No longer!

Let's assume you are cool, clean, and comfortable in your pants and you believe your bike seat is the problem. Saddle discomfort keeps countless women off their bicycles. We think that's a pity because it's the most adjustable factor of the problem.

First, does your bike fit? Are you reaching too far for your handlebars and putting to much pressure on your *mons pubis* and/or clitoris? Is your saddle too high, causing your hips to rock with every pedal stroke and mashing your labia side to side? Assuming your bike frame is close to the right size, try adjusting your saddle. Start with your saddle rails in the middle position on the seat post and with the saddle top perfectly horizontal. Move the saddle forward and aft, or tilt the nose up and down, but only by millimeters at a time.

Tilting the nose of the saddle up will shift weight from your mons and labia towards your bottom, but will cause other problems if you have to reach down for your handlebars. Tilting it down may put more pressure on your hands and cause numbness. You should feel stable in the saddle, with no tendency to slide off and with your weight evenly disbursed. Ride for several miles before adjusting it again. If this isn't helping, the saddle position probably isn't your top issue.

Next, a saddle change-up could make a world of difference. If you're looking for a new one, hard leather saddles and models with a cutout down the center both have their devotees. Many women choose saddles that are much too wide. In riding position, your crotch sits on the saddle, not your butt. A wide saddle can cause even more chafing than a narrow one, rubbing on your bottom and inner thighs. As for softness, be wary. Abundant gel padding tends to squish into places it's not needed, possibly macerating your labia far more than the hardest saddle ever could. If your bicycle and saddle fit well, a very hard saddle might work best. When shopping, remember that some bike shops will let you test ride saddles—if so, take up the offer!

Let's talk now about your shorts and what's in them. Some people cannot stand to ride with any padding at all, for the same reasons that gel saddles can cause problems. For others, padded bike shorts are a comfort upgrade. There are lady-specific bike shorts of varying quality, some with thicker pads than others. Like with saddles, experimentation is the only way to find out what works for you. It is important that your padded shorts are snug; sliding or bunching can cause chafing. Padded shorts with suspenders, called "bibs," stay in place well and cut down on chafing. Some people wear

bike shorts under pants or skirts; keep in mind there are ventilated liner shorts made for this. We strongly recommend you don't wear underwear underneath padded bike shorts. Definitely wash your bike shorts in hot, soapy water after each wear and dry them well so that they don't become a hotbed for bacteria.

The chamois (pronounced "shammy") is the padded part on padded bike shorts. Look for the chamois with the fewest and flattest-laying seams in the crotch area. Using chamois cream helps reduce friction between your skin and your chamois. There are women-specific chamois creams, and ones with anti-inflammatory and anti-infective properties. If you are prone to chafing, slather the cream on your bottom and crotch where it meets your saddle. Then rub some into the chamois. Another line of defense for delicate or angry skin is to rub in a layer of diaper rash ointment with high zinc content *before* putting on chamois cream. Such ointment is protective against moisture and zinc helps prevent and heal infected hair follicles and sores.

Yeast and urinary infections are another common complaint of female-bodied riders. If these infections plague you and you're certain they're not related to soaps, perfumes, prescription meds, wiping back to front, nylon panties, sloppy sex, etc., focus on keeping vulvar homeostasis: cool, clean, and dry on the outside. It's gross to think about, but sweat, the saddle, and movements of riding can cause bacteria to move from the anal area forward. Consider carrying non-antibacterial wet wipes if you're going to be in the saddle a while. Make sure to change out of your shorts immediately after a long or wet ride. And stay well hydrated!

At some point, most of us have freaked out upon discovering alarming pimples and sores. Before you panic about venereal disease, breathe deeply and reminisce on your love affair with your bike. Did you recently have one particularly sweaty or uncomfortable ride? Bacteria thriving in warm beds of moisture, pressure that restricts blood flow, friction, and pubic hair grooming practices that break the skin— all these contribute to skin eruptions. We recommend comfortably hot epsom salt baths, warm compresses, and liberal application of a soothing and/or medicated topical cream (examples are antibiotic ointment, drawing salves such as PRID, benzoyl peroxide-containing zit cream, and tea tree oil compounds). Commiseration with knowledgeable bikey friends will turn up more recommendations. If your saddle sore continues to grow quickly and painfully, and especially if you develop a fever, talk to a doctor instead.

Finally, the simplest and best preventative remedy of all: stand up! Every few minutes while pedaling, stand on the pedals and stretch. Relieve pressure and let air flow. Lift yourself up slightly when riding over major bumps. Allow your legs to help support your weight on the bicycle. Your bottom end will thank you!

We hope we can help make your ride more enjoyable down there, and that you do not hesitate to pass along what you've learned.

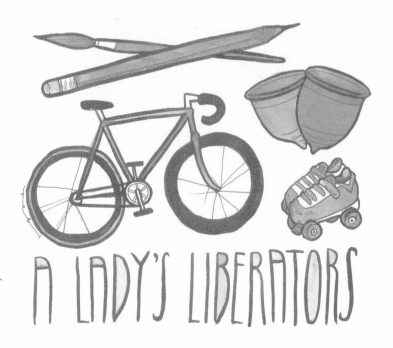

A LADY'S LIBERATORS

THE CUNTRAPTION

Adriane "Li'l Mama Bone Crusher" Ackerman

The Shock Twat's maiden voyage was in 2013 and it was about 10 miles. I left my house in North Portland and pedaled my newly-crafted double-tall bike adorned with a giant papier mache vulva to the Chariot Wars brunch of the annual Minibike Winter celebration of bikes and mayhem.

This bike stands out even in a crowd of other art bikes, tall bikes, and freak bikes. Riding it alone across town, I was wholly unprepared and completely delighted by the responses I got. Lots of honks, lots of face palms, kids stopping whatever it was they were doing and staring as I passed, mouths agape, forgotten hula hoops teetering at ankles, and little minds whirring at lightning speed to try and figure out how they should feel about the giant "naughty bits" that just rolled down the street.

I knew that I would get visceral reactions for sure. But I had spent my time up to this ride mentally preparing myself for the brunch. My main concern was how to convince *anyone* to put their mouth up to the soggy, intimidating tubes that reached out of the Cuntraption, flowing with fermented "blood." I thought maybe I'd have to bribe them with non-pussy wine, or shame them for being vagina-phobic. But much to my delight, from the time I arrived at the brunch through the rest of the weekend there was a consistent line of eager slurpers waiting for their chance to kneel before the giant lady parts and have their throats coated with her rosy flow.

Almost everyone had the same three reactions in the

same order, with a varying spectrum of flare and volume. First, they'd squint or do a little jaw-drop or walk just a bit closer to see if their eyes deceived them. The next reaction would be visceral: grabbing their hair, slapping their knee, turning around in complete disbelief like they were going to walk away, but always completing a 360 as they were drawn back to its sheer awesomesauce. The final reaction was always—*always*—a boisterous laugh or loud exclamation of some sort. (You should've heard and seen the guys on acid. Lordy. It made their year and I'm pretty sure it made them cry).

In only in a small sample of the folks who experienced the Shock Twat did I encounter the rare fourth reaction: The question, "Why?" What could possibly have possessed me? Why would I bring something like this into being? What in the world would make me think of it? I had a rolodex of answers that I'd call on, depending on who asked and how deep I thought they were capable of following me with the reasoning.

What each reaction boiled down to was this: there just ain't enough twat on display in the world, and lord knows I love twat a shocking amount. Pussies are slandered left and right, equated with weakness and with a sense of mystery that is often less than reverent. And yet, in my experience, there are few testaments to a power more striking than hundreds of grown-ass adults waiting in line to get on their knees in front of a giant, hand-made vagina, all for a squirt of boxed wine ... and to feel that for one glorious moment that a giant, inanimate symbol of life, power, and seduction was shining down on them and them alone.

All hail the vulva! All hail the Shock Twat! Viva la Cuntraption!

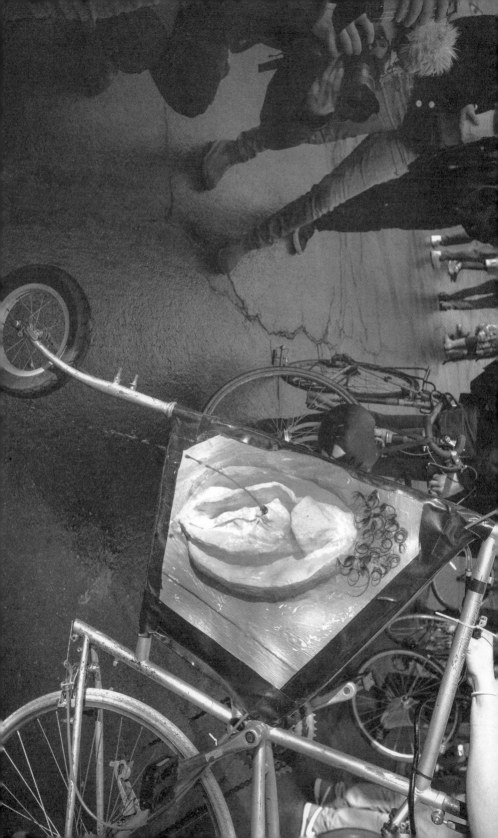

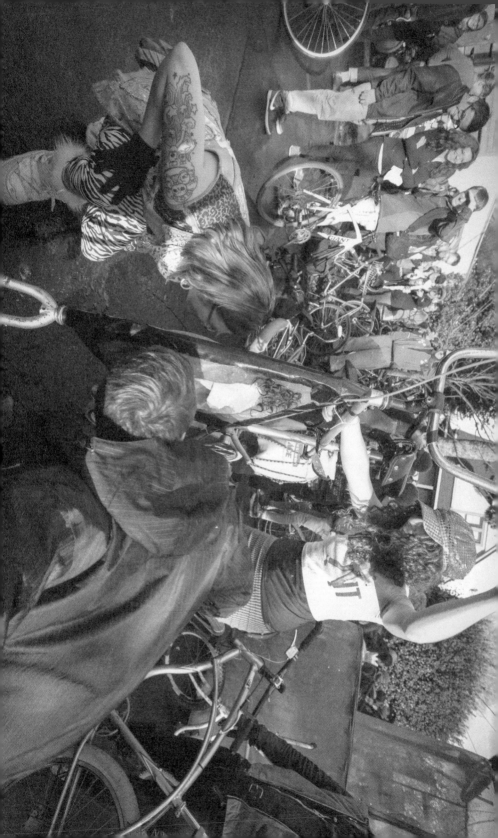

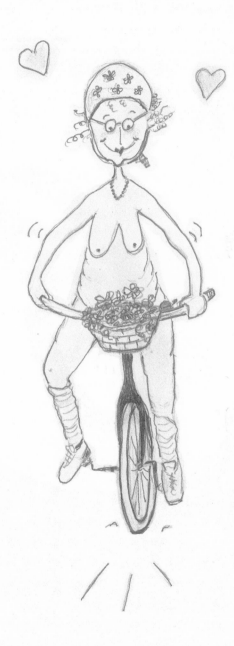

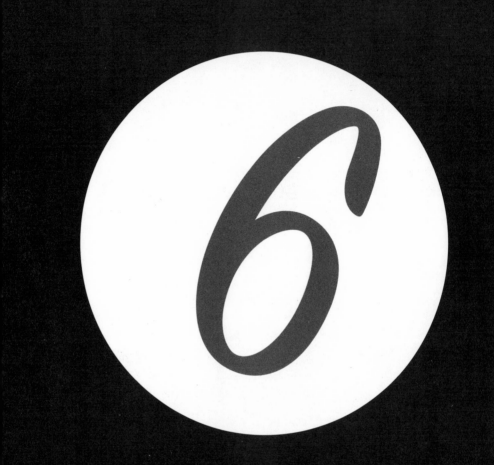

Menstruation

File under: Questions that don't get asked much in bike shops. We love to talk about menstruation and bicycling, because there are in fact specific steps you can take that can make all the difference between cycling comfort and cycling disaster. But it is so rare for anyone to be willing to talk about it at all. Even solely amongst fellow menstruators, it's an embarrassing thing to bring up. Which is, in our opinion, all the more reason to talk about it a lot.

BIKING AND BLEEDING

Elly Blue

For 51% of us, it happens every month, rain or shine, plans or no plans, for decades of our lives. One week we're on top of the world, dashing around with energy, vigor, and aplomb. The next week we might be a little slower, a little hungrier—then we bleed for a few days and the cycle goes back to the beginning. It hits us all differently, and we all deal with it differently. It can be a non-event, a monthly medical crisis, or anything in between. Wherever you fall on this spectrum, here are some tips for riding out your period.

NOTHING BEATS THE CUP

Reusable menstrual cups are a freaking revelation. You insert them entirely into the vaginal canal and they stay in place with light suction. You empty them every so often and carry on about your life. Another benefit is the money you'll save and, over the years, the thousands of pounds of trash you can keep out of the landfills. The most widely available brands in the U.S. are the latex Keeper and the silicone Diva Cup and Moon Cup. But these aren't for everyone—so if you need to go bigger or smaller, or something about the shape or the ridge at the top irritates you, there are a lot of different cups out there with very minor differences—you can buy them online or, increasingly, at the grocery store.

PRODUCT HACKS

I wish reusable pads worked better on the bike. But cotton and wool pads just aren't that great for all but the shortest emergency jaunt to the store—either they are uncomfortably bulky, shift around uselessly, or have a disastrously positioned snap. If these are what you've got, lowering your bike seat a centimeter or two can help keep them from being a major pain in the crotch.

As for disposable pads, the ultra-thin ones aren't terrible for riding. They get saturated with sweat and torn up as you ride, so prepare to change them often.

If you wear tampons, you'll find greater bicycling bliss by snipping that string.

RIDE OUT THE PAIN

If you're prone to cramps or moods before your period, consider getting on your bike and riding somewhere. Exercise is great for reducing and coping with pain, both physical and mental. Even a short bike ride can really turn your day around; and hey, the more pedaling you get in, the better the rest of your month gets too. Other things that can help: Yoga, acupuncture, diet, and taking it easy on the coffee.

SLOW DOWN AS NEEDED

Not everyone gets hit by their period like a ton of bricks, but if you do, slow down and take a break, even if it means staying off the bike for a couple of days. Listening to your body is key—and don't listen to folks who tell you to do otherwise. If bicycling is misery on the hardest days of your period, let that be the justification you need to allow yourself to actually take it easy when your body demands it.

TALK ABOUT IT

Likewise, if you happen to be lucky enough to have an easy period (or none at all), then don't miss a beat by all means—but don't tell those of us who have a bad time to HTFU. Unfortunately, it doesn't work that way. Menstruation is still an awkward topic in most circles, if not outright taboo, and our world isn't set up for folks who feel like death warmed over one day a month. Your friends might get why you'd rather stay in on Friday, but HR certainly doesn't, at least not yet. The more folks who are able to be supportive and actually, you know, talk about this stuff, the better.

SUSTAINABLE CYCLES: BIKING AND MENSTRUATING FROM CALIFORNIA TO NEW YORK CITY

Rachel Horn

I rode my bicycle across the country because it was on my bucket list, but also because I really love my menstrual cup.

I'll save the technical details for you to Google, but in all simplicity the cup is a reusable alternative to tampons—except like way better. I've had mine going on five years, and it still works like a charm.

My beginnings with the cup were rough. First, I had trouble fitting it inside of my vagina. It took time and a lot of troubleshooting with friends to figure out how to use it properly. I had to get comfortable reaching about an inch up there, positioning the cup correctly, pinching it just the right way, and removing it carefully lest it overfloweth upon the floor. It took time and practice, but now it works perfectly. No leaks. No joke.

CUP TIPS

Wash hands before

Wash hands after

Empty sooner rather than later

Insert and remove the cup in the shower to practice

Use only clean water when rinsing

Trim the tail if it's annoying (but *do not* puncture the cup)

Ask a cup-using friend for advice

In 2013, I became a spokeswoman for a project called Sustainable Cycles (.org)—bicycles and menstrual cycles, get it? I biked from San Francisco to New York City, holding women's meetings at stops along the way to talk about about the lifetime waste (300+ pounds), cost (2,000+ dollars), and health issues (dioxins, cotton pesticides, synthetics) around conventional menstrual products. I carried reusable alternatives (cloth pads, sea sponges, menstrual cups) to show and tell, plus a number of cups to gift to attendees. The project provides a refreshing and judgment-free space to discuss periods and how we interact with them.

The bicycle provided a unique—and epic—perspective as we traveled through a dozen states. I zoomed past oppressively tall rocks in Utah, felt the immediate change in temperatures going up and down mountains, internalized the long and dry deserts, and met gracious, kind, generous people. Perfect strangers took us in and gave us countless meals, showers, and shelter—much welcomed surprises after long days of cycling.

Perhaps a bigger surprise, despite the 100-mile days, the 10,000+ foot summits, and steep roads with 15% grades, was my ability to string negative and ugly judgments upon the strong form of my body. I know I am not unique in the struggle for self-love, and only continue to discover the depth to which conventional beauty ideals permeate my psyche. The bike trip helped me recognize the beauty in strength and relentless pedaling. The fact that I used my body to travel 4,624 miles from the west coast to the east coast made me appreciate it all the more. I have come to realize the importance of reminding people how beautiful they are, even if it may seem obvious.

As distinct as they are in form, by the end of the trip I found that the menstrual cup and the bicycle are not so dissimilar in function. Through these possessions, I seize my independence. Independence from spending dollars at the pump and at the pharmacy; greater independence from products like fossil fuels, plastics, cotton, and synthetics that are created by harmful industrial and political processes. I claim

my independence from being stuck in gridlock traffic, and independence from that awful feeling of removing an almost-dry tampon at the end of my period! For myself and for my community, these two simple devices are a step in the right direction.

Famous suffragette Susan B. Anthony once said,

> "I think [bicycling] has done more to emancipate women than anything else in the world. It gives women a feeling of freedom and self-reliance. I stand and rejoice every time I see a woman ride by on a wheel...the picture of free, untrammeled womanhood."

I could say the same of the freedom of the menstrual cup and it would ring just as true.

Sustainable Cycles has more trips planned, loving our bicycles and menstrual cups every stroke of the way—and finding through both a greater strength in womanhood.

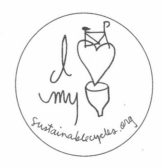

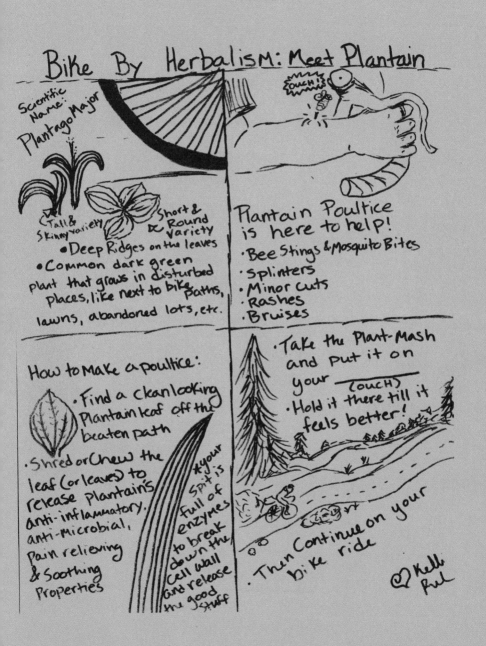

Bike By Herbalism: Meet Plantain

Scientific Name: Plantago Major

← Tall & Skinny variety

Short & Round Variety →

• Deep Ridges on the leaves
• Common dark green plant that grows in disturbed places, like next to bike paths, lawns, abandoned lots, etc.

OUCH!

Plantain Poultice is here to help!
• Bee Stings & Mosquito Bites
• Splinters
• Minor cuts
• Rashes
• Bruises

How to make a poultice:

• Find a clean looking Plantain leaf off the beaten path
• Shred or chew the leaf (or leaves) to release Plantain's anti-inflammatory, anti-microbial, pain relieving & Soothing Properties

*your spit is full of enzymes to break down the cell wall and release the good stuff

• Take the Plant-Mash and put it on your ____ (OUCH)
• Hold it there till it feels better!

• Then continue on your bike ride

♡ Kell Ruh

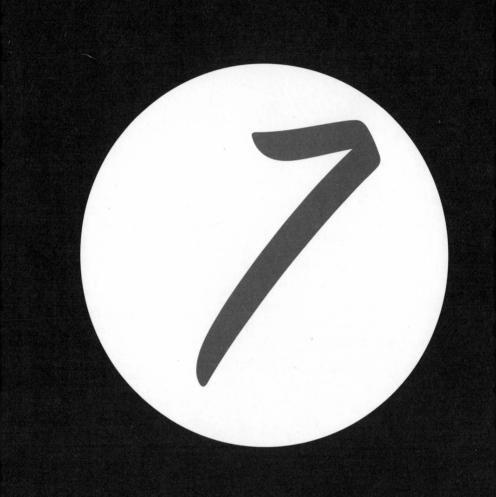

Hot Stuff

There's something innately sexy about bicycling, and there's no reason to let the sexist advertisers and objectification bloggers own the right to say so. When you step aside from the stultifyingly narrow beam of the male gaze and look at the bicycle traffic zooming past, a whole world opens up of beautiful bodies in motion, bright spirits feeling great as they fly by. And forget observation—so much of the appeal of riding a bicycle is the pure pleasure of it, the liberating joy that you have so few chances at in modern life. How can we not compare it to sex, and to feel our own power as sexual beings as we ride?

SEX GODDESS ON TWO WHEELS

Jaymi Tharp

When I ride my bike, I wear short skirts. My legs are strong, muscular, toned, and dead fuckin' sexy. I worked hard for those amazing legs, pedaling miles and miles of my stress and fat away, and loving every minute of it. Those gorgeous stems hold me still as a statue while I track stand at a stoplight. They help me move sexy and slow when I am with my lover. They grab the attention of every motorist, keeping me safe while I speed through my city to the cacophony of catcalls and wolf whistles.

When I ride my bike, I wear spaghetti strap dresses. My arms are steady, lithe, powerful, and carved from marble. I have spent countless hours gripping my handlebars, offering graceful and unerring direction to my steel steed, building layer upon layer of sinewy and inviting curves across my wingspan, fingertips to fingertips. Those arresting arms hold me fast to the road, balanced alluringly above the frame's top tube. They help me hold myself gracefully and enticingly above my lover's face. Pedestrians and motorists alike watch me signal a turn, arm held out yoga-warrior-style in the direction of my intended travel.

When I ride my bike, I hold my head high. And why not? My hair blows in the breeze, catching the wind and the eyes of people glancing through storefront windows. I feel light as a feather, yet my body is working as hard as the well-oiled machine I ride. My face curls into a beautiful smile and I laugh out loud at the beauty of the day and feel it reflected in my face, my body, my self-esteem.

When I ride my bike, I am a sex goddess. I tilt the frame to one side and step over it, my body in the same position to the one I most enjoy when making love. It's sexy as hell. Even on my worst days, even when my voluptuous body is swathed in layers of insulated winter wear, even when I wear a poncho that resembles a trash bag, the sheer power of my bike riding body and my proud, steady attitude make me the sexiest thing on the road.

WHY IT'S GREAT TO DATE A CYCLIST

Anonymous

I'm a cheap date! Bike rides are free.

I think you smell great after a workout.

This pack I carry around everywhere? I'm prepared! If you need a tool, patches, a pump, lubricant... I've got you covered.

You like to shave your legs? I don't judge, just as long as you don't judge me being au naturel.

I think you look sexy in your wool baselayers.

I have core strength, endurance, and *stamina*. These legs and booty don't quit.

When you sleep over I will make you breakfast in the morning because I know how important fuel is to your day.

I love morning rides.

I fully embrace the journey without the pressure of finding the perfect ending. Let's hold hands while we track stand at red lights. Let's hand-sling each other along the Greenway. Let's work our way up some hills and arrive at the top together, breathless.

When you are riding next to me, your cheeks can be red and wind-chapped, snot hanging out of your nose, eyes tearing up from the cold— and I will honestly think you are beautiful.

As a queer person, I get kind of annoyed when people ask me if I'm straight/gay/whatever. When asked I sometimes identify as "bike-sexual." I mostly say that for giggles, but... can you imagine getting into a relationship with someone that doesn't ride a bike semi-regularly? I can't. Bikes make your body fit and strong, you probably have an independent personality if you are into biking around, and considering how much time I spend on my bike I think that being a biker is pretty much a requirement to get into my pants. –Anonymous

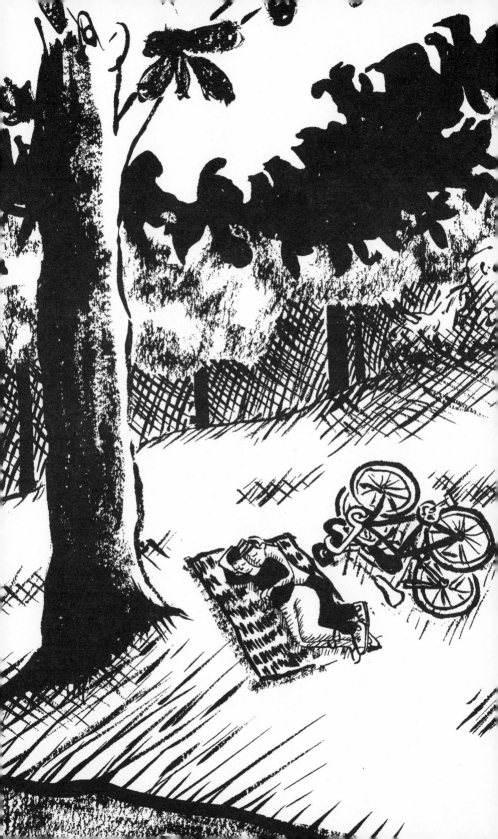

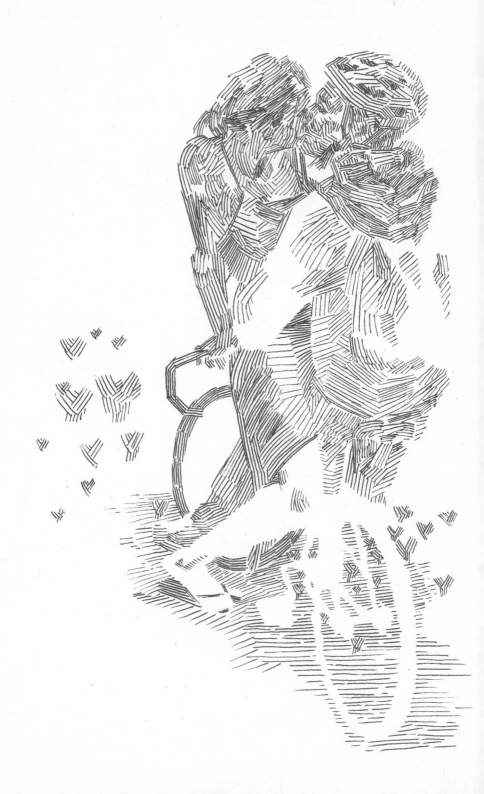

DIVORCE BY BIKE

Josie Smith

I wonder how many people can say that a bike changed their life? I never expected that the desire to prove something to myself—that I could learn to ride a bike—would bubble forth into an adventure of growth and love.

As a child, I had given up on a riding after a few wobbly excursions. Fast forward to age 27. I was feeling stifled by my failing marriage and all of life's other stresses. I wanted to prove to myself that I could do it, ride a bike, and not get killed by a car or my own clumsiness.

So I purchased a homely Fuji hybrid and set out to do it. Starting with the first ride, I felt confident and sure of myself. I felt liberated. I couldn't believe it: here I was, probably the clumsiest person in the world, riding her bike to work and not hitting cars or falling at stop signs.

I wanted to share this experience with my then-husband. I was lonely and wanted to find a way to spend time together. But he wasn't interested in setting aside time to go riding on the weekends. He was tired from his work week and wanted to rest.

I realized the weight I had been carrying for years, of my failing marriage. It had to stop. The vicious circle of our dysfunctional relationship would only end if I became brave enough to say, "I can."

One day I went for my morning trail ride and heard my chain making a rattle of sorts. I had become friends with Travis, the owner of the bike shop next to the trail, and texted him my concern.

He came down the hill like a superhero in a black polo shirt and checked out my bike. It was a beginner's mistake: I had not shifted my grip-shifter far enough. I felt sheepish.

"Do you want company?" Travis asked.

This started the trend of Travis accompanying me at least once a week on my morning bike ride. I enjoyed the lone wolf experience, but I very much enjoyed the company and conversation. I found that riding with someone made it easy for me to talk and be free with my emotions. I found myself filling up with overwhelming and powerful feelings.

I realized my marriage was completely and utterly over. Not only that, but it had been over for at least 5 years and I had been too afraid to admit it. Ending it would be saying, "I failed" or "we failed." It was a big pill to swallow. But finally I was ready to leave. I had to. I was tired of living a life I couldn't thrive in, a life that was holding both of us down and that was never going to feel fulfilling. I had allowed myself the freedom

of having a bicycle; now I wanted to have the freedom of having a healthy and fulfilling relationship.

Divorce is a mental and emotional rollercoaster. There are a lot of thoughts, feelings, and hard realities that you must confront. Realizing that you have found someone you could open your heart to, talk to, respect, and love is a lot to think about as well. It was all very scary and happening simultaneously.

I was starting my life over at 28, ending an almost 10-year relationship and starting fresh with another. Riding my bike salved my wounds, helping me process and deal with all the changes.

My bike really did change my life and it keeps adding so much more to it. I'm finding new passion, new goals and dreams, and the will to make positive changes in my life and the lives of others.

WHEN A SEXY M.F. SNEAKS UP ON YOUR FEBRUARY MORNING

Rhienna Renée Guedry

I was sailing down Greeley Avenue towards downtown on my bicycle, looking out at the city and at the clear day ahead. It was February and it was beautiful. On the southerly cusp of winter, Portland was painted in pastels and gilded with dew. The suggestion of early spring was everywhere—the promise of tiny buds on bare branches, the twelve extra minutes of daylight, the afternoon you biked without gloves and realized your knuckles would not ache from the cold. The gravel and the brown pulp of lingering late-fallen leaves had been swept to the side of the bike lane in a perfect line, like the tide pushing against the shore.

All this bliss, and suddenly this Prince song came on my iPod. But here's the thing: This was a Prince song I'd never heard before. It revealed itself to me like a hidden track, buried eleven silent minutes after the last song on an album, like a B-side or brand-new track that had slipped through my music-collecting floorboards.

"The hell is this?" I asked myself. I liked what I was hearing, or, I should say, my body did. The song made me want to dance up on someone with some serious fervor, to push up against them with one hip, half-lidded eyes, and warm cheeks, and say, "Hay. 'Sup?"

Most cyclists have witnessed their brethren do a kind of pedal dance. These are sometimes reserved for stoplights—hovering like a tight-rope walk to stay perched until a light changes—but others are musical in origin: bike as dance partner *and* dance floor. The rider might rock their hips in time with a secret rhythm, pedal in concert with a beat, nod or wave their head from side to side. Cyclists with headphones or mobile bike sound systems know exactly what I'm talkin' about. I am sometimes this kind of cyclist. You've either ridden behind me and checked me out, or rolled your passive-aggressive Pacific Northwest eyes and pedaled on.

So here I was commuting like any unassuming morning cyclist, listening to this Prince track and, you know, completely turned on. No big deal, right? Except it was before noon, before caffeine, on the side of the road, on my way into downtown. With each revolution of my wheels, I was pushing a little harder into my bike seat than was reasonable, steering my bicycle into tiny lasagna-shaped waves as that Skinny Motherfucker With the High Voice promised me a "touch that makes [me] go insane," to "pull [my] hair, [and] feel no pain," and incredulously/

presumptuously, that "it's about to get freaky 'cause the places that I'll be kissin'/ are the places that no other man could ever find." I may have, unconsciously, bitten my lip. Hard.

Hot damn.

Three minutes and nineteen seconds later, the song ended. The dream Prince of my youth escaped into the purple vapor, and another song began. At the next intersection I caught the light, put my boot down, and caught my breath. I unzipped my jacket at the throat and hit "back" on my iPod to play the song again.

That Sexy Motherfucker.

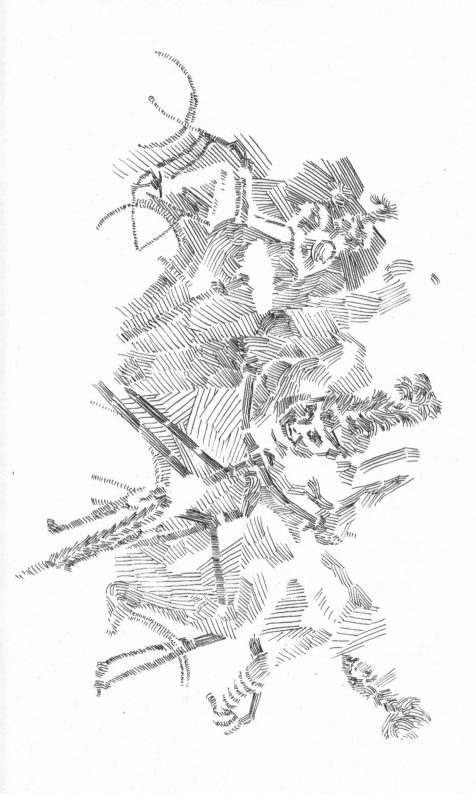

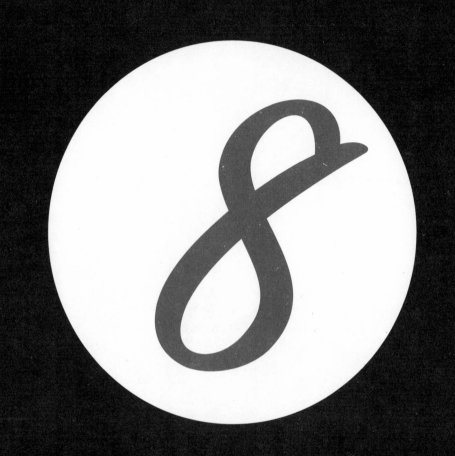

Childbearing

*P*regnancy experiences are filled with commonalities, yet as unique as the babies themselves. The point of this section is acceptance: It's your body, and your experience. We also want to put to rest that that old chestnut that biking is universally bad for pregnant women. Sometimes a bike ride while bulging with a baby-to-be is pure relief. Sometimes it's the easiest way to the birth center. That doesn't mean you have to bike while pregnant, and it doesn't always mean you should bike. It means that, as with every other topic covered in this book, you get to listen to opinion, find facts, assess risk, and make your own choice.

This morning, getting ready to bike to a café across Portland's Willamette River, I was balking a bit at having to go across town through the Cascadian drip and autumnal gray skies. But by the time I had biked for ten minutes and reached the top of the bridge, I felt so alive, with all my blood coursing rhythmically and palpably through my veins. I wondered what my baby was feeling and if it sensed how expansive and connected to everything around me I felt— unshielded, my heightened view in line with the city's outline. On the ride home, even my hand signals felt like primordial greetings without the need for language. Hello there! Turning left. Hello! Goodbye! I realized that because of and in spite of the asphalt by which I choose to commute on two wheels (and for two passengers right now), I get to connect to the world more tangibly. –Monica Christofili

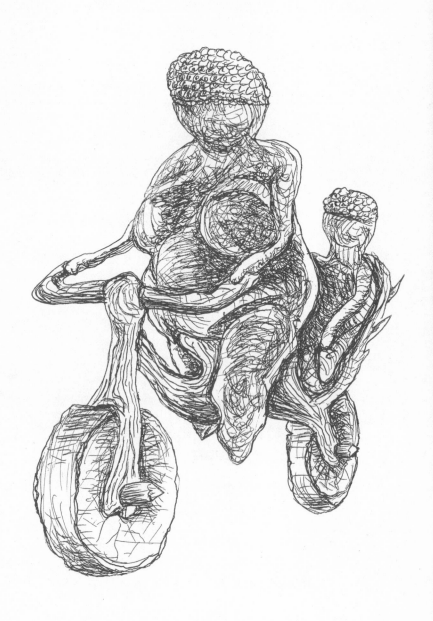

BIKING TO THE BIRTH CENTER

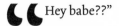

"Hey babe??"

"Yeah?"

"If everything goes ok, I think I'd like to ride to the birth center."

"You sure?"

"I think so. If everything's normal. Yeah."

"Ok."

This little conversation, held at around my thirty-sixth week of pregnancy, might strike some as a bit... insane. While we have no car, neighbors and friends had made it quite clear that they were available day or night to drive us. A taxi had taken me to have my first baby on a sodden Thanksgiving morning just nineteen months before. I saw no reason not to call them again. Nonetheless, at forty weeks and four days I lurched onto my bike at a few minutes past five. Best friend at my side and husband trailing us on the cargo bike with the birth bag, I pedaled through the light chill of the midsummer morning to go have a baby.

My contractions were a little less than five minutes apart. At a mile and a quarter with moderate hills, the ride would take about twenty minutes. That's four contractions to deal with on the road, I reasoned. Maybe five. Easy.

I got on the bike immediately following a contraction, but the next one came sooner than expected. There was no one else on the road. As I felt the sensation crest I breathed deeply, thought about the rotation of the pedals, and spun effortlessly as I let it move through me. Barely a waver. One down.

Two more contractions passed in the same way, and then I

saw the hill ahead. There are bigger hills in the city, but this one was plenty daunting under the circumstances. I stopped at a stop sign, and started a contraction as I began rolling again. I reached the base of the hill just as it faded. Slowly, deliberately, I started to climb. I found my lowest gear. I controlled my breathing. As the road leveled, a fifth contraction overwhelmed me. I wobbled toward a parked car and my friend gasped as I regained my course. And then we were there.

Hey! I rode my bike to the birth center! Should I hurry inside before the next contraction comes or pause for a victorious picture? Pride won out, but barely, and the picture that we snapped bears witness to that next contraction. Five hours later, Kestrel Gayle Proctor came into the world, born underwater, sweet and healthy and ravenous.

I'd ridden my bike throughout pregnancy. I'd toted my toddler around town most days. I'd raced the cyclocross season through my first trimester, battling nausea and fatigue for the chance to get muddy and sweaty in a field of beginner women, laughing and cursing and hauling ass. I'd planned and led Kidical Mass rides, playing mother duck to fleets of slow-moving kids and families as we explored the city and asserted our rights to a place on the roads. So with all that behind me, why not ride my bike in labor?

Barring bad luck, pregnancy is a time of health and vigor. A time that, in spite of incessant hunger or poor appetite or relentless heartburn or weeks of nausea, can be spent fully inhabiting one's body. Doctors and parents and partners stress our fragility and vulnerability, insisting that pregnancy should be defined by a long list of things to be avoided, sacrificed, and feared. They instruct healthy women to "take it easy" and engineer drugged labors or dangerous surgeries. They rob us of a chance to know and embrace our vital power as women. They are the voices of a society that, for all its progress, still views women as weak; a society invested in keeping us from finding our strength.

Like natural childbirth, riding a bike for transportation is not best for all women. For those who need them, I'm grateful that there are hospitals and doctors and NICUs, just as I am glad that people who need cars and buses and taxis to get around can use them. But I'm also grateful that I did not need a hospital to give birth, and I am grateful each day that I don't need an engine to get from here to there. Empowering women to take control of our bodies and our births improves our lives. So does empowering us to be our own engines.

The dominant transportation paradigm robs healthy women of a daily chance to know our physical strength.

The dominant birthing paradigm keeps us from discovering in ourselves the unique power required to deliver a baby. In both cases, the state of "normal" is one that emphasizes weakness: an overdependence on technology to do what we are told we cannot. I reject those paradigms. Riding my bike every day is a choice that celebrates the fact that I can, that I am healthy and strong and fierce. In perhaps this respect only, Kestrel's birth day was no different from any other.

BIKING TOWARDS VBAC

Dena Driscoll

Five weeks postpartum, with a healing fourth-degree tear of my perineum, I carefully climbed back onto my bike and rode with my five-week-old daughter in the outside world for the first time. For most women who have so recently given birth, the thought of riding a bike is likely the last thing on their minds. For me it was a grand finish to my daughter's birth.

A vaginal birth after cesarean section (VBAC) was something I wanted for my second child as soon as I delivered my first. A long labor had forced me into a tough decision; the doctors told me that a C-section was the best way to deliver my son. Exhausted and feeling powerless at that moment, I surrendered my first birth to an OB who used a knife to cut my son out of me in a cold operating room.

Yes, a healthy boy was born. But, as an average, able-bodied woman without any remarkable obstacles beyond a long labor, it was hard to accept that this was my destined and only birth choice.

How does one prepare for a VBAC? I still do not know the right answer. Get tough skin comes to mind. It is a lot like riding a bicycle with children or while pregnant: people will doubt you, will worry about your and the child's safety, and ask far too many personal questions.

For me, strength and planning were important. I found that riding my bicycle while pregnant, with my son in tow, was the invigorating strength building I needed to prepare for birth. I rode until 41 weeks pregnant. Then, after a couple of obstacles at the hospital, I had my long desired VBAC.

The spring day that I first strapped my daughter into my box bike gave me a new feeling of even greater strength. Postpartum, I felt happy in a way that I had not felt with my first. With each slow pedal stroke that spring I helped my body and mind heal. I got stronger with each movement, while my daughter was peacefully lulled to sleep.

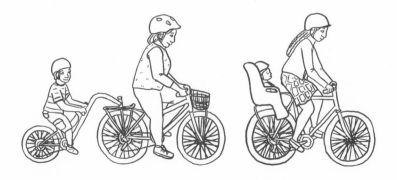

AFTER THE FACT

Katura Reynolds

This is a sad one.

My babies—twins, Alexandria and Edward, a girl and a boy—were born three months too early. Each weighed about two pounds. Too tiny, too fragile to survive. Ed lived for ten days, Alex just six.

This has been a hard year, full of grief, full of a deep struggle to find some meaning in our babies' short lives. But of course, they were alive for much longer than that terrible week in the hospital NICU. When I try to imagine what their pre-birth "memories" of life would have been, I think about the times I felt most alive, and how they must have registered that sensation on some level—our shared triple heart-rates, the endorphins through the umbilical cord. I think of walking, dancing, cycling.

The kids and I rode daily along the forested loveliness of the Ruth Bascom Bike Trail in Eugene, commuting to work with the ospreys and the goldfinches. In Portland, we pedaled the Springwater Trail (clogged with packs of happy joggers) and the Eastbank Esplanade (the thrill of being right down on the river's surface on that stretch of floating path), looking for apartments in the shiny big city. Crossing and crossing the Willamette River, on foot and by bike, the light changing on the water at all times of day.

When they were the size of two pomegranates we went bike camping. Me, always the slow cyclist, now even slower, but feeling strong and steady and happy nonetheless, riding with good friends who were excited by the news of their existence. We racked up the miles on my short, preggo-friendly commute to my new job during the Bike Commute Challenge. We stopped to relish wild blackberries by the roadside on the way home every day. We crept up hills in low gear and coasted down the other side on the way to the library. Slowest bike on the road, for sure. But damn proud.

I miss Alex and Ed terribly. I wish I could have watched them grow up. But if nothing else, I got to share with them a taste of what it feels like to move through the world joyfully, under one's own power. I'm so glad to have had those experiences as positive landmarks around which I can organize my memory of their lives.

CODA

It was a crisp Monday morning, with the pinkness of sunrise still playing on the surface of the river. I perched as a passenger on the back of our longtail cargo bike as my husband pedaled us both downtown. As we waited for a red light, a bike commuter on a fancy fast machine pulled up alongside us and taunted me in a joking way—"That's no fair to make him do all the work!"

"Hey, I'm busy carrying the baby," I retorted, nodding down at my gigantic belly. "We're both carrying passengers here."

Our third child, Margaret, was about to be born, two years and thirteen days after Alex and Ed, our short-lived twins.

It had been a healthy pregnancy and would be a straightforward delivery. The most complicated factor, aside from insurance hassles, was the enormous tangle of mental and emotional hurdles to get through.

I spent my first trimester on foot, teaching myself to play the ukulele as I strolled along. Struggling to learn new fingerings for chords proved an excellent distraction from what could easily have been paralyzing fear.

During the second trimester, I got back on my bike, cycling all over town to prenatal yoga and aqua-aerobics classes. I felt like a badass, daring myself to be more and more active during the same gestational stage that I had spent on bed rest while carrying the twins.

And indeed, I kept riding my bike until the doctor announced that I was one centimeter dilated. The image of having my water break while cycling was just too weird, so I resumed my pedestrian ways. And sure enough, my water broke not long after, while I walked home from work playing "Green Grow the Lilacs" on the ukulele.

Taxi to the hospital, a loaner car to get us all home.

Now I'm learning to walk all over again, with a baby lashed to me in a sling, and wondering how we'll incorporate this tiny new human into our bike routine.

We're so glad of this happy ending, even though the emotional landscape is still complex and unpredictable from moment to moment. Joy and grief are different spokes that blur together as the wheel of life rolls along.

But how can I call it a happy *ending*, when it's so much more of a *beginning*?

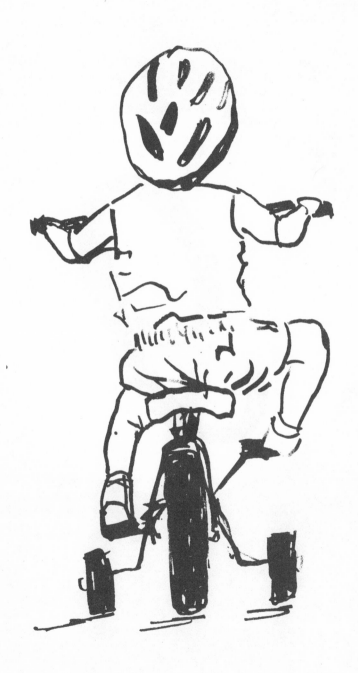

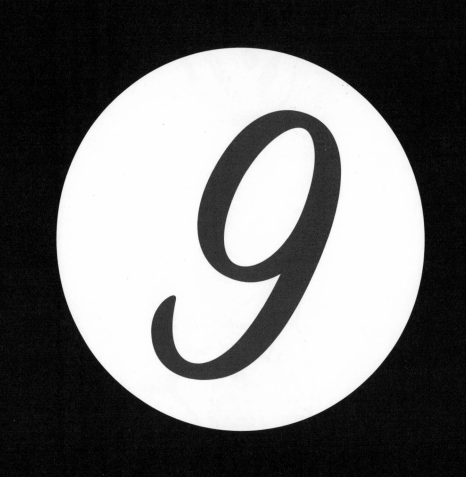

Our Bodies, Our Choice

When we first announced this book, we knew that one topic had to be included, no matter how difficult or controversial it might prove: Reproductive choice. What does this have to do with bicycling, you might ask? Throughout this book runs the question of who gets to decide what it means to be a woman, and also who gets to decide how we move our bodies through the world. One of the major ways in which this control is asserted is using the barriers already built into the landscape and social economy. Clinics closing—and laws that require multiple visits—mean greater distances to travel and more time off work, even just to figure out your options or, increasingly, just to get basic health care. The war against women isn't just about abortion—it's about birth control, about access to knowledge about our bodies, about our ability to move freely, unconstrained by other people's politics and priorities.

CYCLES OF ANXIETY

Constance Winters

I still remember the moment his wife phoned complaining of pains. My cycling companion peeled off in the direction of home, shrugging apologetically for cutting our ride short. It was probably nothing, but you know how these things go: better check in.

By evening, his wife was in the hospital. They discovered a large mass on one of her ovaries. Whether or not it was malignant was not yet clear. But they would find out, they assured him, in the least invasive way possible—so as not to damage The Baby.

The Baby, in this case, was an 8-week fetus. And reading between the lines, it began to dawn on me that the hospital was unwilling to employ diagnostic or treatment methods that might result in its loss.

This turned out to be correct. The following day they announced that they would delay performing a biopsy on the tumor until the pregnancy was further along, so as not to disturb the fetus in its early, delicate stages.

Listening to this account of the situation, I felt a lightheadedness come over me. A knot formed, then tightened, in the pit of my stomach.

Delay performing a biopsy on the tumor... *But what about the mother?*

I wanted to ask this, and at the same time I did not. Because the very fact that no one had mentioned her so far, the fact that the woman's own husband related the doctors' words in the spirit of agreement rather than outrage already answered my question, whether I admitted it to myself or not.

The mother is not the priority. The 8-week cluster of cells in her belly is.

How do I put into words what this realization felt like? It felt like living in a sci-fi dystopia, where at any moment my status of Human might change to the status of Incubator.

It felt akin to discovering that I lived in a country where persons diagnosed with a terminal illness are expected to have their healthy organs pre-emptively harvested. You know, to benefit people with longer lifespans who might need those organs. And that more horrifyingly still, these persons and their families are conditioned to find this absolutely normal. Once diagnosed, the patient arrives at the hospital and, with a serene smile, checks themselves in to have their liver or heart removed. "After all, it's not about me anymore. It's about that other person—

the person with their whole life ahead of them, whom my organs will benefit." The anesthesiologist hovers over their trusting upturned face on the operating table, holding the mask down with a gentle, yet firm hand. End scene...

"If this terrifies you so much, what were you thinking moving over there?" says my friend Karen bluntly. "It's not like you didn't know."

True, I knew about the abortion laws in Northern Ireland before coming to stay here. Back in the US, friends even joked about it nervously. "So...when a woman gets a positive pregnancy test result do, like, alarm bells go off and they come and fit her with an ankle monitor so that she can't leave the country?"

Haha, very funny. But of course (in case you are wondering), this they do not do. Which is precisely why I felt that the abortion issue, in this country of which I am not a citizen, did not affect me and was therefore none of my business. Subjectivity, postmodernism and all that. I was only a visitor after all.

But thinking of the pregnant, tumor-ridden woman who was now receiving questionable medical advice, I understood all at once that it did affect me. Regardless of whether I myself ever "fell pregnant" (as people here so aptly put it) it affected me because it filled me with anxiety over my status as a full-fledged human being.

In my 30s, I find that many of my female peers are entering a phase of their lives where they are trying for a baby. Ten years ago, most of these women would have expressed outrage at the situation in Ireland. Today several of the ones I've spoken with surprise me with decidedly softened views.

"Don't get me wrong, I'm pro choice," says Liz, knitting her brow from the effort of choosing her next words carefully. "But as someone who's been trying to conceive unsuccessfully, I kind of feel like it's not *fair* when women who are pregnant just throw that away ... You know?"

It so happens that I do know. Because, for the first time in my life, I am open to the possibility of having a child... and because, like many of these other women, I am discovering that age is a remarkably effective contraceptive. Being of a generation raised to think of pregnancy as something that would surely strike *the moment a man failed to wear a condom*, it took me some time to adjust to the reality of the situation ... which is, that when a woman aged 35 has sex with a fertile partner, she stands only a 15% chance of conceiving. They did not teach us that part in high school sex ed.

For better or worse, my personal situation has not influenced my outlook on reproductive rights. And my readiness for pregnancy does little to diminish my apprehension of going through it in Northern Ireland. If anything, it only exacerbates my anxiety over being trapped in a dystopian sci-fi. Were it to happen, I would like to spend my pregnancy in this country— because my partner is here and because, in most ways, the quality of life here is excellent. But I am filled with misgivings over the quality of medical care that I (not my fetus, but I—as in *me!*) would receive. Moreover, I do not trust the doctors to tell me whether or not the unborn baby would be healthy (a very real concern, considering my age), and to give me accurate information about its development.

As I imagine the scenario of a positive pregnancy test, already the panic overwhelms me. I find myself frantically planning, scheming, counting months. "If I conceive on such and such a date, I will need to fly back to the US by such and such dates to get all the tests done..." I think of the extra money it will require to do this back and forth dance, about

the stress of travel and being away from my partner, about the uncertainty and chaos of it all. Already I feel like a fugitive. The ankle monitor joke is even less funny than it was initially.

How ironic this all is, when I recall that what originally attracted me to Northern Ireland was the unprecedented sense of freedom I felt when I first arrived. Specifically, the freedom of cycling—the quality and scope of which is almost too good to be true. The endless, glorious back roads with their panoramic views of glens and ocean, the undisturbed wildlife, the "perfect" (well, by my definition) weather, even the presence of like-minded cyclists with whom I immediately bonded. The exhilarating, liberating feel of it all was what lured me in. It is on my bicycle that I feel the most comfortable, the most like myself and the most like the world is limitless— in short, I feel at home. By extension, it was why I felt at home in Northern Ireland even before I met my partner and settled down here.

And now? Now I tell myself that I have to be willing to accept the bad with the good, the proverbial flip side of the coin. So I put money aside in case of unexpected trips to the US. And I try to still the panic that bubbles up within me when I hear updates on my cycling buddy's pregnant wife—updates in which her own well being is seldom mentioned.

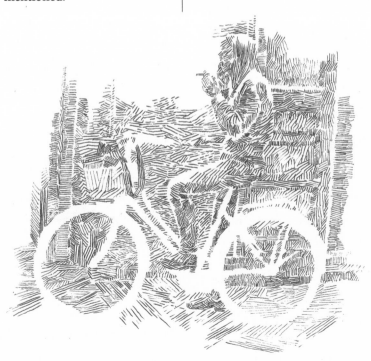

APOLOGIES TO MARGARET SANGER

K.I. Hope

The moon was in waxing crescent, pregnant with light. I slid underneath it, legs rising and falling with my breath, pushing the pedals that pushed me forward. I inhaled the night; this was the kind of bicycle ride that was all sighs, with strong winds and slow strides. The cold wet promise of snow filled my lungs and I struggled against the incline. Less than two weeks until the Full Hunger Moon. Houses still held up their Christmas lights, tiny blinking promises of happier times before December went and the bills came.

Alone on this climb, I felt a pressure deep in me reminding me of my cycle and its bloody ebb and flow. I remembered a sadder time, just before Halloween, when it stopped altogether.

I had met him in summer, and I left him for rain. My two wheels were freedom, but that man was such a force that it took four wheels to carry me five hundred miles due north. I thought of his fetus and gave it some names: I called it "mistake and regret" after a favorite song. I called it little cells that were in me too long. I called it a burden.

I gave him no choice, for it was my decision to make.

Running broken and stiff with the wind at my back, gasping across the state line, I fell safe into Oregon's crooked-branch arms; the sound of coyotes became my alarm. I lived in the nighttime and slept through the day, pushing him out until his scream in my head faded to a whisper. But it wasn't far enough.

I traveled further still, to the last of the West Coast,

where the trees meet the sea. Lighthouses beckoned and I haunted them, pacing the widow's walk and searching for myself.

My girl self was lost, had her voice taken away, floating in the ocean and drowning in regret for not leaving him the moment we'd met. His baby was a snake bite and the vacuum sucked out his poison; without that, assuredly, I would be dead. Pain was the last wound he left, the dull ache of intimacy still his greatest bruise—one no one can see but that always aches, spread black and blue inside to keep lovers away.

I climb on my saddle, I climb on my steed. I pedal off into the sunset, encased in my tomb. The bicycle is solitary. It is the greatest comfort, of reflection and yearning and ache and redemption. Each ride is a victory as I sit on my hips, feeling their width as they span the seat, connecting to my legs and all the good parts of me that are alive.

Each ride is a metaphor for being marginalized. Each car is a man, bigger than me. Each narrow path is another chance to flee. The moon is a woman, wise in her years, beaming on the young as we continue to defy, wearing our wool and soaking it through, leaning far forward and enjoying the view.

I killed something small. And I don't regret it, at all.

TRUE STORY

C.E. Snow

While I am a student at the University of Iowa, I have an unplanned pregnancy.

My car has been sent to a city lot for a parking violation. I have a job as a newspaper reporter and have been getting around Iowa City on a borrowed bicycle.

The bicycle is a demotion. Twenty-five pounds of shame in that college town. I am pregnant, uninsured, carless: irresponsible by everyone's standards.

The Huffy belongs to Beth, daughter of a progressive couple that lets me stay with them. They talk about options. You can have the baby, they say—*you are a newspaper reporter.* Or, don't have the baby—*you're so young.*

I call my parents in Texas to disclose my sin. It's confession, not conversation.

They pull a script from church: I should have the baby because God says that's right. But they will not be supporting my medical costs. They tell me that communication will stop. My sin is too great.

There is this deep hill that drops from the wealthy neighborhood where all the professors live, straight into the Iowa River ravine that borders campus.

I pedal my bike to campus with the phone call rattling around in my head, louder than the wind noise as I bomb down that hill. I apply no effort to the brakes, rolling and rolling, wondering how fast I need to go to break myself.

I am already fragmented.

I seek out a Christian "help" agency that offers medical services, though I soon realize their only goal is to have me put my daughter up to be adopted by one of their miraculous upper class infertile families.

I pore through the binders of families selling themselves to my unborn child and I. The perfect Winnie the Pooh nurseries, the declarations of how I will be so brave to give them my child, how God will surely bless me.

My former roommate is a silent, brilliant stoner named Jake. One day I receive a letter from Jake's mother Inga. The letter includes a check for what I believe is the amount to acquire an abortion, along with pictures of her garden, and a plea:

> "Do not do what the white man tells you to. There is no shame in this, and I will come to Iowa City and sit with you through whatever you choose."

Inga invites me over for meals of duck and Irish coffee. We watch Woody Allen movies together.

Eventually Beth and her Puerto Rican, beret-wearing grandpa help me bail my car out. Then, I pull a fast one.

I drive to Washington D.C., get a press pass and a job at a start up. It's just after 9/11. No one asks about my growing belly. I stay up late at night in a rental house in Falls Church watching *Citizen Ruth* and chuckling to myself. My loneliness turns to solitude.

There's another bicycle in the garage now: a step-through for eleven-year-old Jordan, who divides her time between wishing for longer hair and reading Harry Potter. She wants to know who her grandparents are.

I tell her sometimes adults disagree on how to live. I tell her I was raised by bears.

She doesn't buy it.

We pedal together, slowly, around an inlet of Lake Michigan.

I listen to the perfect, mechanical whirring of our bike chains as we circle the lake. I tell her I appreciate her every day. We brake softly at the intersection, before proceeding.

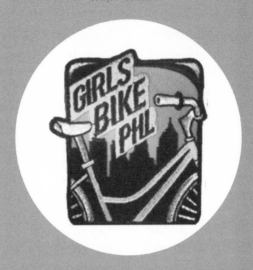

When I turned into Woodland Cemetery on a Saturday last fall, my heart leapt: Fifteen girls, ages nine to eleven, were waiting with their bicycles for me to arrive and teach them about biking. I'm not really a kid person—I normally do bike programming with adult women. But these girls I felt comfortable around.

They were Girl Scouts, and I was there to help them earn the "Girl Scouts on Wheels" patch I had created for Philadelphia. The five-step journey to get the patch takes a Girl Scout through everything from pumping up her tires (the first order of business that day, as some of the bikes hadn't seen the outside of a garage in a while), to safety and handling skills, to mapping routes and exploring her environment.

On that Saturday, we started with a small bike rodeo, moved on to a short ride around the winding roads of the car-free Cemetery, stopped for a snack—Girl Scout cookies, of course—and then set off on a route across a corner of West Philly, ending at Penn Park. As we rode along in a group, the girls periodically screamed "STIIIIICK" or "POTHOOOOOLE" at the top of their lungs. I had asked them to call out obstacles and they got *really* into it! We discovered a beautiful little pedestrian bridge we hadn't known about before. We stopped for water at the top of a hill and felt the wind in our hair as we zoomed down it. That four-mile ride was farther than most of them had ever traveled on their bicycles.

It was a big day for me too. It was the day I realized that "Girl Scouts on Wheels" had gone from an idea I was personally excited about to something that was actually working in the real world. Ten years of experience as a Girl Scout myself plus a few years in the bike advocacy world, and here we were. It was incredible to see the confidence these pre-teens had—even the ones without much prior bike experience were navigating around each other, signaling their turns, and careening down hills by the end of the day. I hope these girls hold onto that confidence and freedom through their awkward teenage years, when girls typically stop riding.

A few weekends after our first adventure, the troop planned and executed an overnight bike trip to nearby Valley Forge Park, pedaling all day on the Schuylkill River Trail to get there.

A few weeks later, I stopped by a Troop meeting to hand out the Girl Scout patches they had earned. My heart overflowed as I distributed them, all the while processing flashbacks of countless hours I'd spent in similar church activity rooms for Troop meetings myself. It was a full-circle moment, one I won't soon forget.

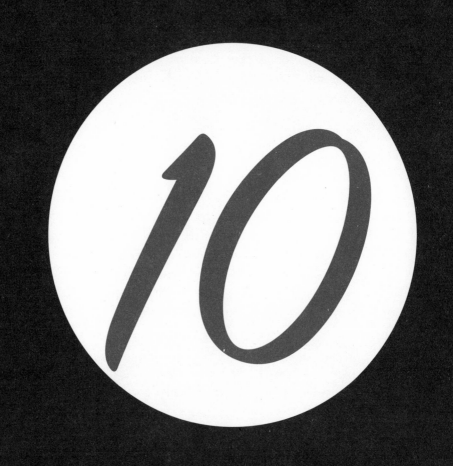

Menopause

From menstruation to menopause a host of family responsibilities can keep women off their bikes. Once the child-bearing years have truly ended it can feel like a lousy deal and a big bummer that hot flashes, a changing body, and brittle bones are the thanks we get. It may seem like the idea of carefree bike riding is only for other women. The 'pause' in menopause is really just another phase in the trajectory of our lives. Finding your way to (or back to) the bike can bring in a new phase of health and wellness, or biking can just be a better, cheaper way to get to the store. Or both. Again and always: Your choice!

AGING BY BICYCLE

Susanne Wright

You might wonder how a 50-something woman fits into the biking world. After all, cycling advertisements resoundingly ignore us. Bike shops, though sincere in their desire to serve the public, don't employ middle-aged women as inspirational role models. You won't find us spread across the shiny pages of cycling magazines or starring in YouTube videos.

Where you will find us, where it really matters, is on the streets of our communities.

I cycle for recreation, fitness, fresh air, and sanity. I'm a member of the Sandwich Generation. Smack dab in the middle of adults aged 40 to 60 who are both caring for an elderly parent and raising their own children. My mother died some years ago and my father's health has steadily declined from the sheer heartache of missing her. I am in charge of his care—from doctor visits, finances, and housekeeping to leisurely visits to help ease his loneliness. I love my father and couldn't imagine any other action than to aid him, but being sandwiched in between the demanding needs of my family and my dad creates a heavy burden. Caregivers get tired, stressed and drained. Caregivers need care too.

I turn to my bike for solace. Out on the road, I allow time, space, and pedal strokes to recharge me. I breathe fresh air deep in my lungs and magically my bike becomes my caregiver, relieving me of weary stress and infusing me with energy and strength. I inhale the fragrance of apple and pear orchards, note the changing colors of the season, and wave friendly greetings to my neighbors. I return home rejuvenated and empowered. Not once has my bike failed to return me to this state of grace. Not once.

My road bike served me well in another way: Menopause.

I naively shrugged off my first hot flash as an odd moment and my first night sweat as a fever. In my mind, I was too young to think about "the change of life" and I successfully ignored all my menopausal warning signs. When I did give it a passing thought, I decided when the time came I'd "Just Say No," like the pithy 1980s anti-drug slogan. I was so successful ignoring the inevitable that when I finally stepped onto a doctor's scale and saw I had gained 15 pounds since my last visit I was in complete shock. In reality, I shouldn't have been. Night sweats, crashing fatigue, and an unmentionable hunger had been increasing in severity for some time. Clearly, I was in denial. But 15 pounds? There

was no denying that. Mystery solved as to why my clothes fit uncomfortably tight.

That day my bike morphed into my sports club on wheels. I was determined to drop those pounds out on the road. Where I live is hilly, with more hills than flats, so finding ascents to grind up wasn't a problem. And grind I did. I sweated and grunted my way to the top of steep inclines, heaving immense sighs of relief on the cooling descents, all the while increasing my mileage until by summer's end I really had left the extra weight out on the road. I had accomplished my goal and it was at that moment that I truly fell in love with my turquoise Trek 2.1. Bought used from a woman selling it to pay her next month's rent, my bike was now the coolest thing ever. It was my therapist and gym. But there was more to come.

My husband and I took our first overnight cycle tour a year ago, setting out to bike around Crater Lake National Park in southern Oregon. Time was limited. We tossed our camping gear in the back of the car, strapped on our bikes, and down the road we flew. Arriving at the park that evening, we pitched our tent, ate our noodle take-out with plastic spoons, and washed it down with warm beer. We fell asleep to the sounds of children playing, the steady drone of motorhome generators, and the lovemaking of the couple next door. We were up at dawn and on our bikes. We rode as the sun came up and marveled as we pedaled around the sheer lip of North America's deepest freshwater lake. We stopped frequently to take in the incredible views and dine on day-old peanut butter and jelly sandwiches from our panniers. With the sun high and hot overhead, we rolled to a stop at a water cascade and eagerly dipped our heads into its delicious cold stream, noting the tiny bright wildflowers that bloomed amid the wet rocks.

Hours later, we finished our ride. We were as satisfied and elated as two hot, sweaty, worn-out bike riders could be. As first cycle touring vacations go, it was regrettably short. Yet it hooked us on a new dream to look forward to—of retirement on the seat of a bike.

BIKING UP TO THE PAUSE: WHAT IT'S LIKE TO BIKE THROUGH PERIMENOPAUSE

Elly Blue interviews Beth Hamon

I ran into my old friend Beth Hamon recently. I asked her how she was doing, expecting to hear about the latest chapter in her shift from bike mechanic to Jewish music performer and teacher. Instead, she leaned in and told me that she's going through an even bigger life change.

Menopause and bicycling is one of the topics that people ask me to write about most often. But even though I'm bound to experience it myself one day, and sooner rather than later, it's something I know scandalously little about—only a vague notion of hot flashes and hormones. It's as though the topic is taboo. But Beth is a candid person, so, for my own edification and yours, I asked her if she'd be willing to tell me about her experience at this point in life from the perspective of a committed bike commuter (and occasional single speed 'cross racer). To my delight, she said an emphatic yes. We met up for coffee a couple of weeks later and she dished the details.

First off, I learned that I've been mistaken for my entire life about what menopause actually is. You aren't officially menopausal until a full year has passed without a period. The lead-up to this point, which can take years and comes with all the interesting physical changes you hear about, is actually called perimenopause. (Or "my friend Perry," as another friend refers to it.)

Beth's about to turn 52 and has been in perimenopause for the past year and a half. Your own experience, she asked me to point out, will definitely vary, depending on your personal mix of hormones and other life circumstances. She also added that men go through similar changes as they get older, though usually their experience is more gradual.

Here are the basic features of perimenopause, as Beth relates them to bicycling:

IRREGULAR PERIODS

Pretty much everyone's period goes haywire during perimenopause, even if their uterus has previously been on a clockwork schedule. For a lot of women, this irregularity is the first sign of what's about to begin. As far as cycling goes, some people might need to start taking measures they didn't have to worry about previously, like resting on the bad days and keeping a stash of ibuprofin and preferred menstrual supplies on hand in their bag or jersey pocket.

VISION PROBLEMS

This one was totally news to me. Apparently many women experience unpredictable bouts of vision problems over the course of perimenopause. Beth told me about two separate vision related issues she has. One is an occasional, disorienting sudden inability to focus her sight—she described it as feeling that "my eyeballs were changing shape." The second, also occasional, issue is "haloes" in the periphery of her vision. For some women, these are just an added edge of sparkle to their field of view; for Beth, they can be blinding. When it happens on her bike, she has to pull over, for anywhere from 5 to 45 minutes. Worse still, they're often followed by a migraine.

MOOD SWINGS

Another classic feature. For Beth, wild, unpredictable mood swings were the first sign of perimenopause. Her period was still regular and the idea of menopause wasn't really on her radar, so she went to a therapist. The therapist asked how old she was and promptly referred her to a doctor. Estrogen replacement therapy can smooth out mood swings pretty well. But, like a lot of people Beth isn't eligible because of other health issues, so she finds other ways to manage. Bicycling is a huge part of this for her. Endorphins calm her moods, "lift clouds of depression," and make the world more manageable to such an extent that her sweetie insists that she go on even just a two mile bike ride every day that she can. Acupuncture helps too, she said, and any kind of personal mindfulness practice.

HOT FLASHES

The most famous character in the perimenopause cast is the hot flash. Beth didn't have much to say on this topic—she said that in two years she's only experienced this once. Fortunately for me, her friend Lynne caught word of this article and sent me an excited email the next day that opened: "For me, the main annoyance is the hot flashes." Lynne is a randonneur and spends long hours on the bike. She's already passed into menopause proper, but still experiences hot flashes every few months. They usually come in rapid-fire succession. Here's how she described them:

"I get hot and sweat, even though it might be cold outside. For me, this is managed by wearing layered wool jerseys and sports bras, rather than synthetics, preferably ones with zippers. I spend the entire ride zipping and unzipping. My head gets hot as well; I have to uncover my ears and the back of my neck to cool down. Hot weather just isn't as much fun; I can only take so much off." While most of her flashes are mild, "Some are pretty overwhelming—they start with a feeling like a mild punch to the gut, and then I'm not feeling particularly functional for the next few minutes. So I slow down until the sensation passes."

BONE DENSITY

Women lose bone density quickly during

perimenopause. "Maybe it's time to stop downhill mountain bike racing in your 50s," Beth said, but otherwise cycling is safe for most women to continue, unless their bone loss is so great that falling poses a major danger. One of the best ways to counter bone loss is to build up strength earlier in life with weight-bearing exercise. Cycling unfortunately is not weight bearing, "but lifting your bike onto the bus rack is!"

FATIGUE

Beth reported that she's tired a lot more now and needs to sleep 9-10 hours a night. Despite the major mood benefits of bicycling every day, there are days when she's just not up to it—or much of anything else. "Give your body a break when it needs it" she told me in a tone that brooked no argumentation. She said that she's stopped racing, which she enjoyed for a few years, though some women are able to continue throughout their fifties. She rides less than she used to—

nearly every day, but just a few miles at a time, adding up to around 2,000 miles a year. "I'd like to ride my bike forever," she said, "but one day I won't want to anymore—either the risk of falling will be too great or I'll just be too tired." She observes Shabbat, not working or doing anything strenuous on Saturdays, and thinks that's a big part of what helps keep her going during the week.

With this, I closed my notebook, head spinning, feeling a combination of dread of my body going haywire in the next 20 years and relief at knowing more about what to expect—and prepare for. "A lot of the stuff they tell you about how to deal with perimenopause is good advice for regular health," was Beth's parting note.

I had jotted down some personal action items in the margin of my notebook. One of them, underlined so hard my pen broke through the paper, was, "keep riding!"

When I saw my first bakfiets, it was love at first sight. If you've never seen one, bakfietsen are Dutch cargo bikes with a box between the rider and the front wheel for carrying kids and their gear. They are 8 feet long and heavy, almost 90 pounds of steel and marine-grade plywood.

I took that first bakfiets for a spin. It was wobbly at first, but I felt comfortable much more quickly than the predicted 10 minutes.

I feared our son would never tolerate it, but we took a chance and put him in the box anyway. He paid close attention while I buckled him onto the bench seat. Then I waited for the inevitable. But there was no screaming, whining, or fussing. No ducking and freaking out like he was afraid something would fall on his head. He was relaxed and seemed to enjoy the ride as we did laps and figure eights in the street.

This could work, I thought. My husband joked that if I could ride the thing home, over the West Hills to our suburban neighborhood out in Hillsboro, he'd buy it on the spot. Then he saw the look in my eye. It would have taken me hours, but I damn well would have done it. But almost $3000 is a lot of money and I hadn't ridden a bike in years. We decided it would be smarter to wait. As a down payment on the dream, we bought me a bike helmet.

We had been carfree for a year, and it worked for us. The double stroller was our vehicle, and we lived near stores and transit. But as we got to know the area, we longed to live closer to friends and activities in Southeast Portland. The next spring we moved—and at the same time a used bakfiets turned up for sale on Craigslist. This never happens, but here was a lovely first-generation model looking for a new home. We bought it and started rolling.

A year later and we have found a tribe of bike friends to ride with and also learned the joy and difficulty of getting around by bakfiets. Our heavy bike is a challenge on hills. I've learned what routes are easier, and to do things like shop at the grocery store that's a bit farther away and uphill so that the ride home is downhill.

My son is seven and has Down syndrome. He communicates in his fashion, but he doesn't talk. He likes to blow raspberries and beatbox along with music. Sometimes he says words, but I don't think anyone but us can understand him.

Every chance to interact with my son, to get to see a glimpse of what he is thinking and feeling, is precious. I can't imagine life without our bakfiets now, because so many of those rare moments of connection happen while riding. We'll say the alphabet together. He'll put his hand on my knee and watch how my leg moves the pedals. He'll look at dogs that we pass.

He loves the bike as much as I do. I know because it comforts him. When we want to go out to eat we pick places that have outdoor seating. If he gets stressed or can't behave we can roll the bike up to our table and he'll happily sit in it while we finish our meal. It changes a situation where we are all getting grumpy to one where we can all relax.

We take the bus to his doctor's office. He doesn't like it, but I can't get 180 pounds of bike and kids up that hill. I realized recently that someday he will be old enough to go to the doctor on his own. Will he drive? I doubt it. He will probably take the bus like many people with intellectual disabilities. By living car-free we have, accidentally, joined him in his world. He will grow up knowing that adults can get around without needing to drive, and that there is no stigma in that.

I don't like all the drivers vs. bikers arguments, the us vs. them mentality. I don't like it when people who are part of the "normal" way of doing things don't allow for the variety of people who live differently in their community, whether by choice or by chance. I look forward to the day that our choice to live without a car doesn't fill our far-flung family with fear the same way finding out our son has Down syndrome filled them with fear. In the last year, my bakfiets has come to symbolize all of this for me.

On a recent ride for ice cream, my son looked back and puckered up. As we pulled away I leaned over the handlebars and gave him a kiss. We couldn't do that if he were in a trailer, or in a seat on the back of a bike, and certainly not if he were buckled into a car seat. A touch or a request for a kiss are such a big deal: They are some of the rare times that he lets anyone see what is going on in his head. I wouldn't trade my beautiful Dutch bike, or my beautiful son, for anything.

Sickness and Health

From chronic illness to scary sickness to the ridiculous little physical indignities of life, there's a lot that can obscure the joys of living and biking. On the other hand, each day alive is a blessing that the bike loves to support—it can be a tonic for foul moods and uncontrollable monkey mind, a preventative miracle, and a low-impact boon for many ailments large and small. For some, the bicycle offers relief from pain and release from immobility; for others, it's a pleasure that must be set aside. The irony is not lost on us how many people are kept off of bicycles for reasons directly related to cars—a debilitating crash, perhaps, or the many conditions that arise from lifelong exposure to air pollution. Other barriers are indirect; when through age, disability, or any number of factors we are unable to drive a car, the roads and developments around us, so convenient in an automobile, become walls around us. In some cases, the bicycle can become a radical way to break free.

WHEELING

Parisa Emam

I didn't expect to trade my bike for a wheelchair at age nineteen. A disabling illness reared its head my first quarter of college and by spring I could no longer stand more than a few minutes at a time. I collected many losses over the course of that year. I quit the Ultimate Frisbee team, quit most of my classes. My heart and muscles and joints quit working the way I expected them to. I stopped viewing my body as active and efficient. I stashed my Trek bike in a garage, its handlebars slowly warping, crammed against a rusty lawnmower.

I grew up on the back of a bicycle. For years my parents lugged my sister and I around in an Equinox trailer attached to their bikes. We'd promptly fall asleep in that yellow cave with our helmets thrumming against the trailer wheels. We loved it.

By age five I held my own on the back of a tandem, powering the rear of my dad's Santana through weekly rides to Matthew's Beach and Golden Gardens in Seattle. He called me his engine. We had our share of mishaps on that bike, to be sure. It launched me from its seat more than once. One crash trapped me under its frame. Its tires once wedged so deep in tulip-field mud that we toppled over and glazed our bodies in mud.

We coaxed that Santana along a cross-Europe expedition and for three weeks rain pounded down our helmet vents. My favorite stuffed monkey clung to the rack, strapped down by bungee cords and camping tarp, its fur forever matted by the downpour. I gathered nuggets of my dad's life history from the rear seat, probing him about his childhood in Iran while I counted the puddles forming in the folds of my purple jacket.

When I got sick, my legs lost their sharp edges and a wheelchair took residence in the trunk of my car. I watched its wheels coat themselves in the tulip-field mud and I didn't wash them clean. I missed riding. My dad plunked me on the back of the Santana again and toted me around the roads near his house, huffing and puffing without my help.

After illness reshaped me, I thought about buying an electric bicycle. When I floated the idea by an acquaintance, he asked if I instead needed help learning how to shift gears properly on a regular bike. I soon learned that snide remarks abound when it comes to motor-assisted riding, usually from other bike enthusiasts. At the time, I couldn't articulate what riding meant to me or what it would mean to grant myself access to that freedom again.

The day I brought home my red electric bike, my lungs re-inflated on downhill coasting wind. I wound my wheels around the one-block park beside my house until my calves earned enough muscle to tackle waterside roads and trails over old train track beds. My body revealed its fearlessness, balanced atop tires that bucked and hurtled over obstacles.

I added my electric bicycle to the garage three months ago. As illness redefines my body, I must continually redefine my requirements for an accessible bike. It turns out nothing supersedes the agency that comes from propelling my own body through space. Sometimes in my sleep, I whip down the evergreen trails again. My brain dreams up bikes as mutable as my illness, ones that shift and grow with me like appendages. And in daylight, I give in to my passion for riding over any preconceived expectation of how a bike—or a body— should perform.

"YOU'RE TOO PRETTY TO BE DISABLED"

Halley Weaver

Sweaty and disheveled, my back aching from an old injury and a day of lugging around my crap, I drag my bike up to the front of the bus. Every movement is an agonizing effort. Unhinging and lowering the rack without dropping it seems a mammoth task. Hefting my road bike up into the back slot, tiny as the steel frame is, aches my bones and creaks my frame. When I lift the arm that secures the wheel, the spring resists as if locked back against itself.

Task complete, I finally gather my bag and get on the bus, showing the bus driver my lanyard with its permanent Honored Citizen card. The bus driver smiles, the crow's feet in the corners of his eyes wrinkling in cheery joviality, framed by his snowy muzzle of a beard.

"You're too pretty to be disabled," he quips.

I smile meekly, a girlish blush rising in my cheeks as I take my seat.

Internally, I felt slapped in the face. I could preach for the next ten stops about the lack of thoroughness of his company's sensitivity training to people with disabilities. I could tell him volumes about "invisible" and "sitting" disabilities.

If chronic back pain were the worst of my problems, I might not feel so hostile. With only that, life would be a basket of lactose-free, gluten-free, egg-free, banana-free cupcakes.

Really, I am a pretty optimistic person. I don't walk around wearing a bright pink shirt saying, "I Make Epilepsy Look Good." (Actually, I did make that shirt once, but I digress.)

I thought back to ten years ago to when I lived in Boston, riding the train with a friend who is legally blind as well as epileptic. Not being a Massachusetts resident, I paid full fare. She showed her Honored Citizen card and experienced less pleasant treatment by the conductor. She didn't fit the profile of what a visually impaired person should look like. She was wearing make-up. She was dressed nicely. Her hair was styled and colored.

Being "legally blind" and being "totally blind" are completely different things. She can see to some extent. But because of her visuospatial issues including epilepsy (which is how I originally met her), she is unable to ride a bike. So when she came and visited me a couple of years ago in Portland, I had the opportunity to take her to a human-powered vehicle meet up. She was able to try steering a few recumbent tricycles with some success. Instead of using the bus for her entire stay, we borrowed a recumbent tandem. While she had no experience or muscle memory for pedaling, being able to share my passion for cycling with her was really special for both of us.

To me cycling means freedom.

Some days I wake up and feel like utter shit warmed over. And those days suck. Those are the days I rely on other people to ferry me around from Point A to Point B by their personal vehicle, or else I take the bus. Or god help me, a taxi.

Better days, I bicycle. My wheels are my wings to fly—I don't have to rely on anyone else's schedule.

That particular day was a good day that turned into a bad one—I ended up too exhausted to make the six-mile summer evening bike ride home. Yet just a month later I organized a charity ride where I guided four other cyclists over 100 miles with

almost 3,000 feet of elevation
gain in 80 degree weather.

If I looked pretty on the bus,
I must have looked fucking
beautiful on the bike.

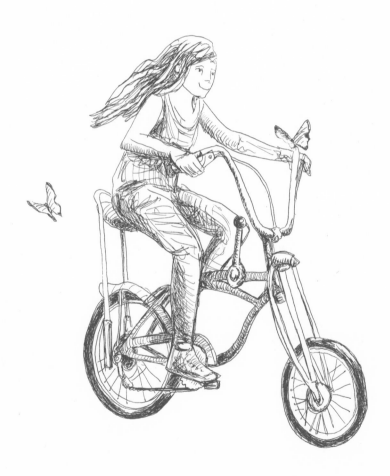

CARS DID THIS TO ME

Lisa Sagrati

For over ten years, I was a hardcore, car-free, transportation cyclist. Bicycling enriched my life in many ways: I met my partner and lots of friends through Critical Mass and bicycle advocacy, I got into fantastic physical shape, I became a much more confident person, and I was able to work part-time because I didn't have to support a car. Working part-time was especially good for my mental health. It allowed me a slower pace of life, with time to study and do unpaid community work.

But at times, I wondered if bicycling in our car-centric society might be harming my health—at least my mental health. I didn't need coffee to get going in the mornings like my co-workers did; I had my morning ride. But by the time I arrived at work, my nerves were often as jangled as if I'd downed a gallon of coffee.

There are some cyclists who can cruise through traffic, calmly bending the rules to their own advantage, wearing earbuds, blissfully unaware of the drivers around them who are steaming up their windows in fury. I was not one of those cyclists.

Riding on the streets caused me almost continuous stress. Although I believed that cyclists had the same right to the road as drivers, I knew the frustration that results from being trapped in a slow-moving car. Whenever drivers were unable to pass me on a narrow street, I could feel their impatience. In response I felt defensive and apologetic for taking up space and slowing them down.

I knew how I needed to ride to keep myself safe—out of the door zone, away from curbs, taking the lane on narrow streets—but all those principles of effective cycling force drivers to slow down or move over to pass.

I felt constant strain from my need to ride assertively combined with my feeling that asserting myself meant inconveniencing and angering others.

I had stopped driving a car when I was 22 because I saw it as inherently violent, alienating, and out of touch with natural human speeds and rhythms. I did not want to participate in that kind of culture. But I found that when I biked in traffic, I pushed myself to ride as fast as possible, trying to keep up with cars and deter drivers from passing unnecessarily—which never worked. I felt driven by drivers—and by my own anxieties.

In woo-speak, I had weak boundaries. But to a certain extent, that's beside the point. I may have been more sensitive than some other cyclists, but that doesn't excuse the drivers who went out of their way to make my commute as difficult and dangerous as possible.

I began biking for transportation in St. Louis. Like most Americans, St. Louisans think of bicycles as recreational equipment and roads as exclusively for the use of cars. It's a working-class city where attitudes are slow to change. I found that nonconformist behavior like riding a bicycle for transportation often made me a target of abuse. This ran a spectrum from relatively mild harassment, such as aggressive honking, yelling, or giving me the finger, to more dangerous threats, like deliberately side-swiping me, throwing things at me, and trying to startle me. These encounters left me rattled and seething for hours or, in the more frightening cases, for days. When someone intentionally threatened my safety, I felt violated, powerless, and outraged. I hated that the abuse and reckless endangerment of cyclists was more or less normal in our culture, and that I had no legal recourse against my attackers. Strengthening my emotional boundaries might have allowed me to go about my business without worrying so much about other people's feelings, but how could I ever adapt to people invading my personal space with high-speed heavy machinery?

Occasionally I was able to catch up with someone who had buzzed me and vent my anger at them. That gave me some satisfaction, but the stress of confrontation was almost as unsettling as the stress of being assaulted.

Eventually, I felt afraid every single time I left the house to go somewhere on my bicycle. My body was operating under a burden of constant stress and anxiety, almost anytime I went anywhere, for ten years.

In addition to the people who played games with my safety were, of course, drivers who were simply oblivious—they weren't looking for bikes on the road or were unaware of how much room they should leave when passing a cyclist. These people were easier for me to accept intellectually, since their behavior was not malicious, but a near miss was a near miss as far as my body was concerned.

A friend of mine in St. Louis gave up his car when he became a Buddhist monk and began riding a bike instead. Soon after he started riding, he was struck from behind by a pickup truck. Although he was not injured, he quit biking and only walked or took the bus for transportation after that. He prioritized his mental well being and physical safety over any ideological commitment to bicycling.

Not me. I kept going.

One reason I persisted was that I was addicted to the aerobic exercise. Walking, even for long distances, just didn't give me the same endorphin rush as biking. But my primary motivation was my belief that bikes are the most efficient, practical, ecological, economical, and healthy mode of urban transportation. I believed in bicycling. But beliefs are for brains, not bodies. In my mind, I felt like one of the tiny minority of Americans who are "strong and fearless" about cycling. But my body was firmly in the majority "interested but concerned" camp.

As any natural medicine practitioner will tell you, our bodies are not designed to handle prolonged stress. We have a fight-or-flight mechanism that gives us surges of hormones to deal with sudden threats, which we all need when we're avoiding predators on the savannah. But natural rhythms include plenty of downtime. Constant stress can rewire a body's circuits into chronic hypervigilance, which can deplete the adrenals, wear down the nervous system, and damage the immune response.

Which helps to explain why my physical health collapsed four years ago.

I had long dreamed of moving to Portland. I believed it would be a bicycling utopia compared to the Midwest, and in 2008 I finally was able to move there from St. Louis. It was a joy to see so many other cyclists on the street and the culture of driving was markedly different. Most

drivers expected to see bikes on the streets and treated me with courtesy. But Portland remains a North American city, dominated by car culture. Many of its attempts to accommodate bikes on the road were half-hearted and ill conceived. The city painted bike lanes too close to parked cars and to the right of right-turn lanes, giving cyclists the choice of riding in a dangerous position on the road or breaking the law and angering drivers by riding to the left of the bike lane. Facing that daily choice wasn't much better than riding in a city without bicycle infrastructure.

The overall vibe in Portland may have been a lot mellower than in St. Louis, but I still encountered plenty of anti-bike sentiment and occasional harassment. One scene stands out in my mind. My partner and I were headed home after buying bread at the Dave's Killer Bread outlet in Milwaukie, south of Portland. We saw a minivan several hundred yards ahead of us about to turn onto the road from a driveway. Although there was no other traffic, the driver waited until we were almost at his driveway before pulling out right in front of us. Then he stopped, forcing us to brake suddenly. He rolled down his window and began spewing an anti-bike rant. Ignoring him, I passed him on the left and continued on my way. He passed me without moving over, his car a foot away from my body.

It wasn't too long after that incident that I became ill. It was as if my body said, "We moved to Portland and we're still going to be terrorized by haters? Sorry, but I've had enough."

.   .   .

I've been disabled for most of the past four years. On January 30, 2010, my stamina mysteriously vanished. Biking and walking even short distances became dangerous, as I could end up bed-ridden for days, too exhausted even to sit up and drink a glass of water. Mild exertion caused me severe muscle and joint pain, unlike anything I'd experienced before. Living in an attic apartment, I was housebound for long periods, too fragile to manage the stairs.

For most of those years I did not have insurance, which limited my access to mainstream medicine. The most doctors could tell me was that there were problems with my immune system and my cortisol production. The best diagnosis they could come up with was Chronic Fatigue Syndrome, a murky condition with no known cure.

Shortly after my ACA insurance became effective, I saw a doctor at a specialty clinic. He diagnosed me with Lyme disease. I resisted the diagnosis at first. I had no memory of a tick bite. I hadn't been in the woods for months before I became ill. But as I learned more about Lyme, it made more sense. Lyme is tricky; it can hide from the immune system. It can lie dormant in the body for long periods, emerging when the immune system is weak. It attacks us where we're most vulnerable, making existing problems—like weak adrenals—worse.

And since I began treatment for Lyme, I've gotten my life back. I'm not 100% better yet, but I can bike and walk moderate distances without fear of collapsing. Proof enough for me that the diagnosis was correct.

I'm not blaming cars for giving me Lyme disease. But I am blaming cars for wearing down my health, slowly, over many years, weakening my immune and endocrine systems, leaving me more vulnerable to serious illness.

.   .   .

My illness was a valuable experience. Chronic illness *will* transform a person— it can make you bitter and resigned, or you can use it as a wake-up call. Over the past four years, I have developed a much clearer sense of my purpose, more compassion, and stronger boundaries. I've addressed some very limiting emotional blockages, and I've gained a sense of spirituality. I spent the last two years of my illness retraining my nervous system by practicing the ancient Chinese art of qigong.

It's gentle exercise, a far cry from sprinting to catch green lights and biking centuries. One of my teachers defines it as "the art of developing trust between body and mind"—a trust I betrayed for many years.

It's challenging work, breaking down old, maladaptive patterns. But we can cause great damage if we neglect this work. Car culture is stressful and unhealthy for everyone, not just for the people outside the cars. Getting around without owning and driving a car should be an option for everyone, not just for the brave or the stubborn. Until we begin to be honest with ourselves about the true costs of driving, we will all pay its price.

EVERY BREATH

Jacqueline A. Gross

I.

I was on my honeymoon in October 1998 when I started coughing. My partner and I were sitting in our room at a bed and breakfast in Cambria and I coughed. Once. Twice. I didn't think anything of it; maybe it was allergies, or an early cold. I live in the Bay Area and with the changeability of our weather, almost anything can happen. I took some cold medicine and we finished our trip in high spirits.

A week later, I was still coughing.

My eyesight took a turn towards the bizarre as indistinct shapes appeared in the margins of my vision. But it was intermittent. I told myself I probably needed new glasses. I ignored the growing fatigue and the loss of appetite, putting it all down to being tired. However, the creeping sense that something was really wrong wouldn't budge. Everything came to a head when I lost my sense of taste at Thanksgiving and tumors appeared over both of my eyes.

At the age of 35, I was diagnosed with respiratory sarcoidosis. The treatment involved high doses of prednisone coupled with loss of control of my body. The feeling wasn't new: Two years before I had a cardiac catheterization to fix a problem with my heart, followed by an ACL replacement on my left knee.

My late thirties felt like a litany of my body's failings.

As I approach 50, I reaffirm my faith in my body by the rise and fall of my pedals.

II.

When I was a kid, I was chunky. Pleasingly plump was a more polite way of saying the same thing: I had a body that some did not think fit with the world around it. When I look at pictures of myself from that time, I see round brown cheeks and a wide smile. Plump, yes.

At my all-girl's Catholic school, I was insulated from some of the slings and arrows that plagued other girls my age. We played kickball on asphalt, scraped knees and hands in our quest to get the opposing player out. At home, I rode my bike.

My first bike was blue and white and came from Sears. It had a white basket with plastic flowers firmly attached to the front. Once the training wheels came off, I went up and down our suburban street, my legs pumping as fast as I could go. I envied my brother's Spyder with its high handlebars and sparkling blue seat. That was a bike that could take you places, or at least around the block, which was still a mystery to me.

That's what bikes were/are about: Getting you to where you want to go; solving the mystery of what's around this block and then the next.

III.

I found my way around the block, graduating from my true blue two-wheeled companion to a yellow Ross Eurotour 5. Eventually, when my father's Raleigh Record passed into my hands, I began a love/hate relationship with its Brooks saddle, which had been shaped and molded by two butts before mine. I learned how to ride without hands, leaning back just-so to keep my balance and giving off an aura of what little bit of cool I possessed.

My brakes went out one day as I flew down a hill by my house. A curb served as a convenient stop and the grass acted as a rough landing pad. I lay on my back staring up at the sky, mentally checking myself for damages until a neighbor stuck her head out of her front door to see if I was still alive. My weak wave assured her that I was in no need of an ambulance.

IV.

A lifetime and a few bikes later, I now ride an upright. My partner inherited my previous bike after years of ill-disguised lust. "I've been waiting for you to upgrade," she said as we picked it up from the bike shop after it had been retrofitted for her. "Are you sure you don't want a new one?" I asked.

She didn't. She likes the frame and the look. We ride together when we can, though my longer legs mean I might lose her if I forget to slow down.

I monitor my body with an eye towards a possible relapse of the sarcoid. When I ride, it is with the knowledge that the damage in my lungs is as much a part of me as are my creaky knees. I draw the air in as deep as I can and let it out, feeling the strong and steady beat of my now-fixed heart.

V.

Coming back from a ride one morning, I slowed to let a man and his son cross the street but was surprised when he waved me on. As I passed by he shouted, "Yeah, keep it going! Keep the momentum!"

I waved at him and picked up speed, rounding the corner so I could head for home. Legs pumping, heart beating.

I smiled.

Yes.

MY BICYCLE IS MY SECOND DOCTOR

Beth Hamon

I spent a rather mobile childhood riding my bike all over my various neighborhoods in Pennsylvania, California, and Oregon. By the time I entered high school, I was riding to and from school nearly every day, a round trip of about six miles. This was in the late 1970s, after the oil crisis had ended and everyone had gleefully gone back to driving—except me. I loved the freedom and ease of bicycling so much that I put off getting a drivers license until my twenties, and by the time I was 30 I'd decided to live car-free (or at most car-lite) for the rest of my life.

I also spent most of my childhood making sure I knew where the bathroom was wherever I went: the mall, the beach, the grocery store, my school. I developed a sweet, innocent disposition that would melt the heart of the most hardened shopkeeper so I could use the restroom. I assumed it was normal to have to go to the bathroom many times each day and simply lived with it until things got so bad that I could not eat without experiencing great pain. I went to the doctor and asked for help. It took weeks of tests and more pain before I got an answer.

The culprit, I learned in my early 30s, was Crohn's disease, a hereditary autoimmune disorder that made my body think last night's spaghetti was actually a deadly pathogen to be attacked and defeated. While I was relieved to finally discover the reason for a life spent largely in public restrooms, I was saddened to learn that my condition was incurable and that I'd likely need daily maintenance medication for the rest of my life.

I would also need surgery, which I undertook in late 1999 to remove part of my digestive path—a common result of the disease. While I recovered in the hospital, the doctors told me that all that bike riding had made me a much better candidate for surgery than most Crohn's patients and had helped the surgery go more smoothly. More importantly, they also urged me to keep riding my bike once I recovered. While no western doctor would come right out and say that daily exercise would ease the effects of Crohn's disease, they all told me that exercising was far better than living a sedentary life, if only to help move the overload of toxins through my body faster and more easily.

Bicycle riding has helped me to stay physically healthier and much more mentally positive about living with Crohn's—and living in general. I could not get health insurance on my own for many years; with a chronic condition, bicycling was the best health plan I could have. I made a conscious decision that if I couldn't afford health insurance or a retirement plan, I would live a life that let me be as physically active and as healthy as I could be for as long as possible.

There are days when I am too fatigued to ride very much. That's a part of living with the disease, as I cannot fully extract all the nutrients from my food and my body expends a lot of energy trying to fight my food. But with the combination of drugs, a carefully monitored diet, vitamins, and all that bike riding, I know I'm doing better than I would be if I'd resigned myself to a sedentary life and had just given up. My daily bicycle riding also gives me endurance, muscle tone, and what my GI doc calls the "glow of health." People who meet me for the first time are surprised to learn that I live with a chronic illness. I don't look like a sick person.

In 2006, I set a goal of riding 2,000 miles, which I accomplished by the first week of December. I've since averaged between 2,000 and 2,500 miles a year, mostly just by riding my bike for transportation, but also dabbling here and there in cycle touring and even racing. Riding my bicycle is a big part of what keeps me physically healthy and mentally calm and happy.

I can sit and moan about the dreadful state of health care in this country—and it is dreadful, make no mistake— or I can embrace the things I *can* do about my life and health, and keep on riding my bicycle.

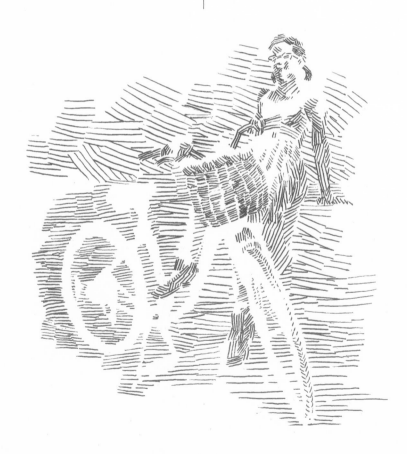

BIKE-ABILITY

Sarah Rebolloso McCullough

I came to bike activism, like many, without much thought as to how my bodily ability privileged me. I reveled in my strong legs and steady lungs. Bicycling was a way to celebrate and enliven the potential of my body. It made me feel free and capable.

Ability is a complicated thing. I speak of ability as the physical, mental, and emotional capacities required for functioning in this world. Because of the world we create, some people's bodies come to be classified as disabled. They are often marked in some way, seen as separate and different from others. Meanwhile, those whose abilities align well with the dominant world can enjoy an existence where able-bodiedness is assumed. It becomes an invisible privilege.

Freedom of choice is central to both bicycling and reproductive rights activism—to choose to ride and to choose the destinies of our bodies. But this framing can leave out those with disabilities. To explore this dynamic, I relate my own experiences within the bike movement and draw upon the work of disability rights activist and feminist D.A. Caeton. (1)

FREEDOM OF CHOICE AND BIKING

Many involved in bicycling activism and advocacy want to make bicycling open to as many people as possible. The growth in conversations around bike equity demonstrates this commitment. And yet, it is still difficult to talk about how those with disabilities fit into bike movements, and often end up ignored.

Celebrating the freedom of the bicycle rolls off our tongues, as does joyful expression of the independence of car-free living. They can become unquestionable goods. And yet, these values can be tricky. They are not easily accessible to all bodies, and they are expressions of privilege. These feelings of freedom and independence only come if we are able to access the technology of the bicycle.

Instead of beginning with the assumption that we are all independent beings that can come together if we choose, what if we assumed that we are all already interdependent? After all, we all depend on technologies and other people all the time in our daily lives.

To enjoy bicycling, we also must depend on transportation infrastructure, good or bad. With good infrastructure, we feel safe while riding. This sense of safety allows the happy feelings riding can produce to grow even more. This means that our feelings of freedom and independence rely upon our relationship with a machine and the environment around us. The way we feel relies on the world we build.

Disability rights activists are very aware of this dynamic and of the bad feelings produced by living in a world that is not made for your body and its accompanying technologies. This is why they

smashed curb cuts into the sidewalk, protested public transit accessibility, and demanded the passage of the Americans with Disabilities Act. We depend upon good infrastructure in public space to accommodate our mode of moving about the world.

FREEDOM OF CHOICE AND REPRODUCTION

In the reproductive rights movement, the needs and desires of those with disabilities are also often overlooked. So many conversations focus on the right to choose, implicitly the choice to not be pregnant. But what about the choice to conceive? And what about the rights of the disabled to live? Caeton points out that the right to choose can often work against the survival and reproduction of an entire class of people with disabilities. He quotes Georgina Kleege, "People take for granted that I don't have children because I don't want to reproduce my defective genes. Who would want to risk bringing a blind child into the world? On two separate occasions in my life, women have told me that they would abort a fetus if they knew it would grow up to be blind." To assume that people with impaired eyesight have a lesser human value is offensive and a potential infringement of their rights.

Often, those with disabilities must fight for their right to reproduce. Widespread, involuntary sterilization still haunts recent memory. Choice does not have to only mean the autonomy a woman deserves over her body. It can also mean the decision to enter into a relationship of interdependence.

In talking about reproductive choice, the focus is most often on the pregnant body. But what about the broader relationships of interdependence upon which reproduction and fostering life rely? Could we reframe reproductive rights such that it also encompasses the right to live, or even thrive, beyond the moment of birth? Such an interdependent approach would also demand resources that foster life throughout its development. That means resources for new parents, good and affordable childcare, safe neighborhoods, livable wages, accessible health care, and all the other necessities for reproducing a good life. It would mean recognizing reproduction not as an independent event, but a choice hinging on our relationships with each other and the structures of the world.

Let's build a dialogue about feminism and bicycling that includes the concerns of people with disabilities. This won't necessarily be easy. It will require those of us who are temporarily able-bodied to recognize our own privilege and how the world is made for us. It will also require many of us to question our feelings of independence and freedom. In exchange, we will get more equitable movements and, when we succeed, a world in which everyone at every point in life can move freely and feel empowered rather than constrained by our connections with each other and our infrastructure. We can relish our interdependence as a solid site for building solidarity and recognition of our differences.

(1) D.A. Caeton, "Choice of a Lifetime: Disability, Feminism, and Reproductive Rights," *Disability Studies Quarterly* 31:1 (2011)

THE PHYSICAL AND MENTAL VICTORIES OF CYCLING

Kristin Eagle

In the past, anyone would easily have called me a private person or even a loner type, keeping to myself. I'd never quite felt a part of any groups or communities. My whole world changed after I was diagnosed with cancer. For the first couple of years, I kept this news so quiet that only my family, doctor, and a few close friends knew. I did not feel comfortable mentioning the topic to anyone else. I was also motivated by fear. It's hard for a shy person like myself to come out and start sharing my fight with others.

My opinion slowly changed as I got deeper into the cycling community. I was relearning to bike in order to help fight my cancer. And as I did, I started coming out of my protective shell. I let a few more people know my situation and what drew me back to bicycling.

Some of the people I told were concerned and didn't agree with my cancer-fighting tactics of cycling and change of diet. But other

people responded with so much encouragement and excitement that I was simply blown away. People wanted to help me on my rides, teach me better ways to tackle hills, and share in my fears, pain and triumphs. Wow.

For someone who kept to herself most her life, this was truly touching. Suddenly, I started feeling more courageous to talk about having cancer. I started wondering if there was any way I could pay back the community for their support by sharing my adventures. I didn't want to only target only other cancer patients; I wanted to help everyone discover a deep inner passion to get on a bike or to keep riding. Everything I have learned from and shared with friends and family has helped me to keep fighting and believing in the power of humanity.

Cycling is good for your health. You don't need to be hardcore or obsessive about it. Just get on a bike fairly regularly, and you'll learn so much about yourself. You'll discover how strong you already are and how strong you can become, and you'll get to enjoy how mentally exhilarating bicycling is. And if you allow yourself to get to know some cyclists, you'll also discover an incredible community.

Three years into my fight, I started my own cycling website, VeloHut.com, hoping to share what I've learned about myself and about cycling. I didn't know where it would go or where it might take me, so it was a complete guessing game as to what I would be doing with the site. When asked who would be the audience, I said, "bicyclists."

"What kind?"

"What do you mean?"

"Race? Road? Mountain?"

"Bicyclists," was my only response. I was laughed at numerous times. To me that meant a challenge I now had to tackle. I don't care what kind of bicycle you ride. As long as you're riding, trying, and enjoying yourself, you're ok in my book. Hogwash to the idea that I had to target my site to one type of rider.

Men, women, kids, teens, elders, road, mountain, BMX,

trike, unicycle, tandems—VeloHut is for anyone and everyone who loves riding a bicycle. To those out there that said it wasn't possible, I say: Open your mind. We are all part of the bicycling community and I believe in the power of our passion and ability to share and guide each other.

VeloHut is built around the people I've met and have come to respect. It's in honor of all of them. I'll keep pouring my heart and soul into it in hopes that I can continue to grow the site. I dream that at some point I can have a strong enough voice to make an impact on the bicycling community and infrastructure. Most of all, I want to share the voices of my newfound friends.

Over the last five years, I've learned that I'm not alone. There are so many people out there cheering me on. I have enjoyed cheering them on at the same time. I used to think the Strava "Kudos" was just silly. Now I love giving people a pat on the back. Everyone's victories and triumphs are different. I'm honored and thrilled to be a part of such a healthy and lively community.

A LICENSE TO BIKE

Synthia Nicole

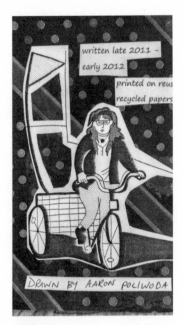

written late 2011 - early 2012

printed on reus recycled papers

DRAWN BY AARON POLIWODA

I have had my road bike since 2002. Man, I fell in love with it right away. When I was diagnosed with anxiety and depression shortly afterward, I refused medication. I biked the 5.4 miles to work, which totally helped the anxious tendencies and being hard on myself. It was so empowering!

But. A blood vessel exploded in my brain in June 2004. I had three brain surgeries in a month. I don't recall the week before or a month and a half afterward. Some of my cerebellum was removed and other parts of my brain were affected as well.

And—my driver's license was cancelled! It was the least of my worries then.

For a while I was in a wheelchair, then a walker. I bought a five-speed adult tricycle, which was delivered in a box. A former partner came over and put it together in a few hours. I could have used a two-wheeled bicycle, but I felt more comfortable with the tricycle.

Frustrating times on the tricycle: I took up more room on the streets, using a slanted sidewalk was no fun, and I wasn't able to go as fast. I bought a 'Slow Moving Vehicle' sign and my dad bolted it to the back of my basket. I also had a flag and some reflective tape. It felt odd to wait at a stoplight without my feet on the ground.

Yet, this tricycle brought the groceries home. Once I laid a blanket in the basket, tied my dog to the basket, and went down to the Minneapolis greenway. He propped himself up with his tongue out, wind in his face.

I moved from the Minneapolis to a small town of 14,000 in order to be less cognitively bewildered. I just don't make decisions as sharply post-injury. That's a difficult one to admit.

I am doing pretty good most days. But my post-injury body utilizes itself much differently, and adjustments—mental, physical, and emotional—seem continually necessary. I have constant, chronic pain in my hamstrings, but the spastic pain is much more manageable after a Botox injection, 12 lumbar injections, and becoming chemical-free.

Most of the time there is acceptance and appreciation for this vessel—my body, my vessel.

I wanted to bike to work so I bought a city bicycle. I lay out my route beforehand. It has felt really good.

Yet, when it's cold—well, I'm not a year-round rider and public transportation is only available from 6am to 5pm, Monday through Friday. So I finally passed my behind-the-wheel exam in August. It was a freedom I didn't know I would enjoy so much. It had been just over ten years since I'd driven a car independently. I'm pretty excited to have this type of transportation available again.

Then—another shift. Back to Minneapolis. A great spring day—perfect to do a few errands with my city bike. But I debate taking it out. I'm hesitant. It has been quite a while since I've ridden a two-wheeler on the city streets.

Then I decide it's going to be now or who-knows-when.

My ride is great. Yes, difficult at times—I have to stop when checking over my shoulder, I can't do that while pedaling.

On the way home, I can feel my thigh muscles working. I'm stoked to have made the trip safely.

I think I'm gonna be okay.

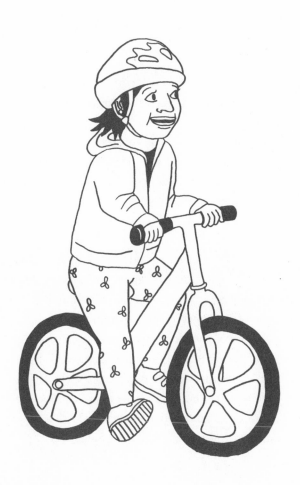

I didn't own my first car until I was in my late 20's. I had ridden my bike everywhere since I first left home to move across the country to a little town in Montana I'd never heard of. I still hadn't wrapped my head around the idea that I could have some kind of mental health issue. I wasn't depressed; I was just having a rough week, or month, or several months. That wasn't an anxiety attack; I just got a little too excited over whatever was going on. Whenever these things would start to become more than just little black rain clouds—when they would thunder and roar—I got on my bike.

I only recently took note of the fact that I have spent years caring for my mental welfare by riding my bike. All those times when I've felt myself going batshit over something that I normally would just shrug off, I've gone on a bike ride to clear my head. When I simply can't find motivation to do anything productive, I've ridden my bike to the video store for movies that, after my ride, weren't needed anymore. When my feet were too heavy to lift, I let my pedals lift them for me.

The simple rhythm of pedaling and breathing, the fresh air, feeling my heart pumping and reminding me that *I am alive* has been my medication for years. So has the amazing community of people who ride together, share together and care together. Trying my best not to get hit by a car is a welcome distraction from whatever is rolling around in my head. Being in touch with my body and feeling all of its healthy potential, as well as finding new challenges—namely hills—pushes me to continue to look ahead and focus on positive goals. Before I ever admitted, even to myself, that my depression was a real thing, my bike has taken care of me.

Now, being fully aware of my mental disorder and how instrumental riding my bike has been in managing it, I am much more assertive about using this amazing tool to its full potential. I'm in my 30s now and can accept that I have had this issue for a long time. Therapy and medication have added their stock to the pot now, too. They help me to maintain the motivation to take care of myself. On really bad days, I find the longest, easiest ride I can and just let my negative thoughts get lost in the rhythm of my pedaling and my breathing. When I start to feel anxiety peeking out, I find the biggest hill I can and put all of that energy and emotion in a healthy place.

That deep burn in my thighs after a long ride and the chicken-legged walk the next morning remind me that I did something worthwhile and that I'm worthwhile. I don't feel beat up, I feel like I beat something. On my bike, I found a way to put my anxiety and depression in their place.

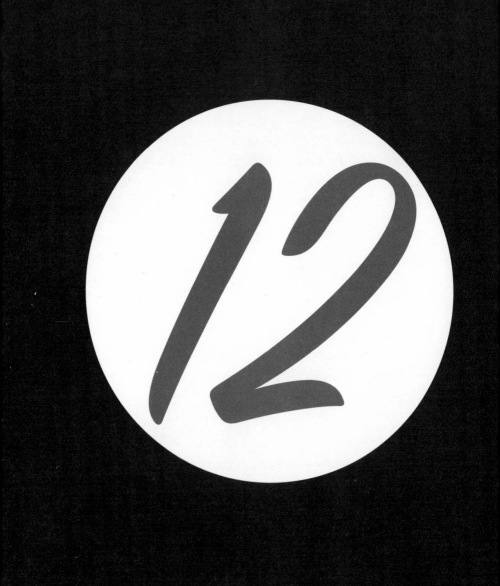

Sports

*D*oes bicycling to the grocery store have anything in common with bicycling on a racetrack? The bikes are different, the clothes are different, different roads are used at different speeds and with different habits of stopping (or not) at intersections. The cultures, attitudes, and advocacy goals often seem worlds apart. In Dutch there are even different words for the two activities. Increasingly, though, we meet people for whom the sport of cycling—be it a racing habit or participating in a fundraising ride—is an entry into the everyday logistics of getting around town by bicycle.

In the United States, unlike the Netherlands, our bicycle transportation culture is hugely influenced by the reality that cycling has been primarily viewed as a sport—a men's, elite sport—for much of the last century. Even purely transportation riders like we are can't escape it: The concerns of the sport side of riding have become our concerns, and its pitfalls our pitfalls.

Yet some of the best changes to how we view the two- (or three- or four!) wheeled, human-powered machine are coming from inside the sport of cycling. The idea of equal prize purses for mens' and womens' bike racing events was laughed at five years ago. Now it's a fast-spreading trend.

Hopefully this final section contains the inspiration and resources you need to build the necessary next steps, whatever they are, in your life and in the world.

EQUAL PAY FOR EQUAL WORK

Julie Gourinchas

The UCI (*Union Cycliste Internationale*) is the international body that regulates bicycle racing, setting the rules for where and when races take place, for who qualifies to race, and for other standards like prize money and drug testing. At the UCI World Championships in 2011, UCI president Pat McQuaid incited an avalanche of controversy after his comments in response to demand that professional women cyclists be paid a minimum salary for their work. He stated that "women's cycling has not developed enough that we are at that level," triggering infuriated responses from prominent female cyclists.

Ina-Yoko Teutenberg of Germany said, "I think that's total bullshit. We've seen in the last number of years that it's getting more and more professional. [...] I don't know why guys would deserve a minimum salary and women don't. We're living in the 21st century so there should be equal rights for everybody."

Even more notable was Chloe Hosking's now famous response: "What can you say, Pat McQuaid is a dick."

It is true that women's professional cycling is a younger sport than men's, since women were barred from racing in the early years of the twentieth century. Women's cycling has been neglected in part because of society's pervasive mindset of internalized misogyny and the repercussions of comments like McQuaid's.

I discovered an interesting phenomenon while researching McQuaid's misogynistic commentary. All my search terms focused on McQuaid. "Pat McQuaid women's salary," "Pat

McQuaid women's minimum wage," etc. But the large majority of the results focused on Hosking. These results were not even about her initial statement, but rather the apology that many commentators felt she owed McQuaid.

Which is all the more ironic, given that women's cycling receives a far inferior amount of media attention than men's. Hosking hit the problem head-on: "To say at the biggest sporting event for women's cycling that we haven't progressed enough to have a minimum salary—how do we progress if we all have to still work and we can't support ourselves?"

It's not really a secret that, when compared to their male counterparts, female cyclists enjoy much less coverage and pay. This is not an issue exclusive to cycling. In 2012, the Women's Sport and Fitness Foundation found that "women's sport only received 5% of coverage and 0.5% of commercial sponsorship."

While making further statements about the state of women's cycling, McQuaid continued to deftly dodge the topic of equal pay via minimum salaries. When he ran for re-election in 2013, part of his platform included: "[ensuring] quality in cycling through the development of women's cycling."

Surely, equal pay and the development and quality of women's cycling go hand in hand. The lack of a minimum salary necessitates that women cyclists, unlike their male counterparts, work other jobs. Without the salary, many female cyclists simply do not have the time to dedicate to improving themselves in the sport.

It becomes an awful chicken/egg problem. Not enough money = no way to build quality = not enough money. It's not for lack of interest, though. When ESPN's X Games decided to award equal prize money to men and women in 2009, female participation skyrocketed.

If we take McQuaid's words at face value and accept the notion that women's cycling has not made enough advances professionally to warrant a minimum salary for its athletes, then we can also use McQuaid's words against him. For if women's cycling has not progressed enough, then what is he, as president of the UCI, planning to do in order to advance it?

Women's professional cycling has made progress in leaps and bounds in certain niches—cyclocross, for example, was the first sport ready to offer equal prize money to its world champions, and its popularity has grown tremendously since this decision.

Instead of continuing to starve women's cycling by claiming it is not popular or exciting enough, it seems McQuaid should put up equal pay minimum salaries and

watch to see how popular it could be.

Editor's note: Since this piece was written, McQuaid was voted out and a new guy, Brian Cookson, was voted in, partly on the promise of increasing the pay and profile of women's professional cycling. In 2014 a group of top professional women cyclists formed a pressure group to work for fair pay and full participation in the Tour de France, among other demands. Cookson replied by suggesting incremental changes instead. He said that it was "too soon" to institute a minimum wage for professional women. Instead, he proposed making women's races longer and harder in order to make them more interesting to watch.

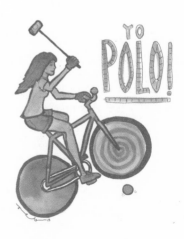

ASS NEBULA

Kristen Rudberg

"I'm pretty sure you should know the bruise on your left cheek now looks like an ass nebula," my boyfriend says, eyeing me from behind as I struggle to squirm into my bike shorts.

I sigh, resigned. A few days before, it had been classified as a minor galaxy. Seems like my bruise has ideas of its own.

I'd already suspected the bloom on the bruise had spread, its tentacles undulating across my derrière like a very slow, very drunk octopus. Or as my boyfriend put it, an interstellar object on the move.

I can feel it every time I sit down. I feel this one, as well as the many others scattered like distant stars across my body. They're linked together, not by the inexorable dance of gravity but by the recent punishing sport I've taken up. A sport that scares the living shit out of me and makes me feel incredibly humble. A bike sport called cyclocross.

As with all things I engage in without adequately considering the implications, these bike races have me furiously wondering—in the middle of racing, no less—*what was I thinking?!* I hyperventilate at the start line, my heart and lungs competing to see which can accelerate fastest. When we finally start, I'm last out of the gate. My only mantra is, "Try not to die." All thought of self-control is out of the window. I alternate between wanting to cry and wanting to throw up. I fall over and over again. I fall in sand. I fall going over a log. I fall in mud, in water, on hills and under dales. I fall on other riders. In short, there's a reason I've got the night sky in bruises littering my body.

Why you ask? Why? Yeah. I've been thinking about that.

At first, it was just a suggestion from my boyfriend. One day he causally mentioned that racing 'cross looked like a fun way to spend the fall. I thought, why not? It can't be that hard. I researched the sport on the Internet and it looked like the majority of people drank massive amounts of beer and rang cowbells 'til the cows came home. I thought, really, this is a sport?

I thought that up until my first race, when I lined up in the beginner category. I was surrounded by women who were in incredible shape. Most were obviously longtime road racers, and only qualified as beginners because they were just now getting into 'cross. I discreetly and meekly melted into the back of the pack.

That first race almost killed me. As a rule, I don't like being noticed and I prefer to be in the background. So it was with particular horror that I rounded the second lap and heard the announcer call my name and number. I wanted to shrink into the ground and completely disappear. By that time, I'd fallen about three times. On the fourth fall my bike seat twisted so hard I had to forfeit the race. I was secretly thanking every God who ever existed for getting me off of that godforsaken course.

As I was trudging off the course, looking properly dismayed at my "bad" bike seat fortune, a gentleman with a giant foam hand asked why I was quitting. I motioned to my bike seat and he said to me, "Aw man. We were really rooting for you!" I mumbled a thank you. He said,"You know what? I think I can fix that!" He strode up to my bike seat and with one good wrench and one giant foam hand, got it back into position. My Good Samaritan then motioned me back onto the course. I could have killed him.

I finished. I was worse for wear and with the first round of many bruises appearing on my elbows and thighs. I bought a lifetime supply of arnica bruise cream, gingerly crept into bed that night, and woke up the next day feeling like a tattered rag doll.

And then ... and then. I began noting my bruises and their migrations with curiosity. My friends demanded to see them, evidence of my indomitable spirit or insanity or both. Soon they became painful, grudging badges of honor. As the season went on, I kept showing up at races. I breathed easier at the start line, I fell less often, and I was eagerly looking forward to races. The crisp fall air, the outrageous fans, the combined happiness and intensity of the spectators—all of it blended into an exciting, incredible way to spend my time.

I still had the bruises. I still had the lifetime supply of arnica cream. But at the end of the season I checked the expiration date on the cream—it should last me through next season too.

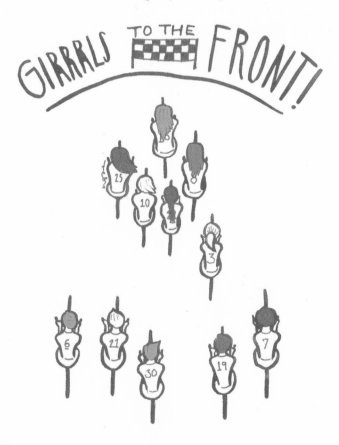

HOW TO BE FAST

Lindsay Kandra

1 DECIDE WHY YOU WANT TO BE FAST

"Fast" is a subjective term. Do you want to take an hour off your best century time? Win a cyclocross race? Know that you can get to work on time if you leave the house ten minutes late? The goal dictates the training.

2. RIDE FAST

Yes, ugh, training. Only a select few extraordinary humans are naturally fast on a bicycle. The rest of us mere mortals have to cultivate our speed through training.

If you want to get fast, be prepared to introduce yourself to the interval. Put simply, intervals are timed efforts at a given intensity level. These efforts can vary in time and intensity and will include brief periods of recovery in between individual intervals or sets of intervals.

Intervals not only condition your legs for speed, they also condition your heart and lungs to perform efficiently during the efforts and recover quickly between efforts.

Intensity can be measured using a few different standards: perceived rate of exertion (PRE), heart rate, or power output. When you first start out on the "fast path," the perceived exertion scale is a great tool that doesn't require any special equipment. It simply means measuring the level of effort your body is putting into pedaling on a scale of 1-10.

To give you an example of interval training, here is a workout I use when teaching indoor cycling for cyclocrossers and short-course triathletes:

1.   10 minute warm-up at PRE 4-5. Don't do an interval workout without warming up for at least 10 minutes. This prepares your muscles and

pulmonary and respiratory systems for the workout.

2.   Three sets of the following sequence: 3 minutes at PRE 7-8, 1 minute rest, 2 minutes at PRE 8-9, 1 minute rest, 1 minute at PRE 9-10, 1 minute rest, 1 minute at PRE 9-10, 1 minute rest, 2 minutes at PRE 8-9, 1 minute rest, 3 minutes at PRE 7-8. At the end of this sequence, rest 3-5 minutes before beginning again.

3.   10 minutes of cool-down, followed by a full body stretching session. Cool-downs are as essential as warm-ups. A cool-down helps your body flush out the toxins that you produce during the hard efforts, thereby decreasing post-workout muscle soreness.

During an interval workout, there are a few ways to switch things up: climbing out of the saddle, pedaling at a higher cadence, or doing 20 second "pushes" of increased efforts in the middle of your interval.

Many racers do their interval workouts on stationary indoor trainers to have a controlled, traffic-free environment to work out in. You can always take your workouts outside, but note that it will be harder to control your efforts when you factor in weather, road conditions, available daylight, and traffic.

3. RIDE SLOW

This may seem counterintuitive, but you have to be willing to ride slow to be able to ride fast. There are two ways bike racers incorporate the slow ride into their training regimens. First, during the off-season we ride slowly to help our bodies recover from racing and to build an endurance base for the upcoming season. Second, we ride slowly during our race seasons to help our bodies recover between interval workouts or after races.

Many new racers think they have to ride hard during every workout in order to get faster. This is a common mistake. If we ride hard each and every time we get on the bike, we are neither rested for quality interval workouts, nor ready when it really matters—on race day.

4. GET STRONG

Fast bodies are strong bodies. For that reason, many cyclists incorporate some sort of strength training into their regimens. That you would need strong legs to be fast is a no-brainer, but having a strong core and upper body is also essential. If your core and upper body are weak, you waste energy holding your body upright that could be used to power your legs. You also risk straining your back and shoulder muscles during hard efforts.

Strength training can take many forms. Traditionally, it has meant a weight room with free weights. But if this isn't your style, functional strength classes (CrossFit is a popular example) or vigorous types of yoga also provide core and muscle conditioning benefits.

5. REST

Recovery is hands-down the most frequently ignored component of training.

In order to complete your interval workouts at their intended intensity and be fresh on race day, you need to be well rested. This means getting enough quality sleep and taking sufficient time to recover between hard rides.

Rest also means listening to your body during a workout. It is one thing to abandon a workout or skip a ride because it is "too hard," but it is another to call it a day because you are sick, sleep-deprived, or stressed. Your body will thank you during your next workout for the extra rest.

SECRETS OF CYCLING SUPER POWERS

Emily June Street

Two activities in my life make me feel like a superheroine: Pilates and cycling. When I'm soaring on a descent, I consider how Pilates allows me to unleash my bike-flight superpower. On a bicycle—as in life—my strong center lends me balance and confidence. This core strength allows me to pedal smoothly and comfortably, without injury-provoking compensations in the hips and back.

Pilates is a conditioning method invented by Joseph H. Pilates in the early twentieth century. He called his method *Contrology*, the science of moving and breathing precisely and fluidly. It has become well known for its core-strengthening benefits.

Pilates has much to offer any athlete—I consider it my secret edge in many physical endeavors—but it is appropriate even for a casual cyclist.

The starting point for any Pilates exercise is the center, though the ultimate goal is to develop uniform strength and flexibility throughout the body for efficient, powerful movement in a full range.

You can start Pilates—and enhance your superpowers—with a few simple exercises. Here are five of my favorite mat exercises to get you going. Use an extra thick mat (half-inch or thicker) so you do not bruise the back. Perform each movement five to ten times.

ROLLING LIKE A BALL

I love Rolling Like A Ball because it stretches and massages my back after longer rides. It also refines internal balance perception—

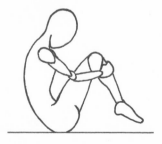

vital for any form of bicycling or superheroics.

1.   Begin sitting with bent knees.

2.   Hold backs of thighs (easy version) or fronts of shins (harder) and tuck the hips under to find a balancing point where feet lift from the ground.

3.   The back should be rounded like the letter "C."

4.   Looking at the navel, suck the belly in and roll backwards to the shoulder blades with a deep inhalation.

5.   Avoid throwing the head back.

6.   Exhale completely while rolling back up to balance on the tailbone.

7.   Use the abdominal muscles to suspend in this balanced position for a moment before repeating the roll.

ELBOW-TO-KNEE

Side belly muscles are the secret behind most superpowers. Elbow-to-Knee strengthens the oblique abdominal muscles, which play a crucial role in stabilizing the torso during cycling. They help prevent the body from lurching side to side, a common problem during climbing or intense effort. This exercise also teaches how to hold the pelvis still while bending the hip joint. Stable hips keep the lower back happy and maximize leg power

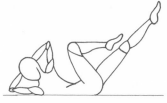

1.   Begin lying supine on the mat. Bring knees towards chest so the feet lift from the ground.

2.   Support the head and neck with hands behind the head. Curl up, drawing the navel in towards the spine.

3.   Extend one leg out at 45 degrees to the ground, keeping the back of the hips firmly on the mat.

4.   Bring an elbow across to the opposite bent knee

by twisting at the waist and increasing the curl upwards.

5.   Switch and repeat several times, inhaling for two switches and exhaling for two switches.

6.   Avoid rocking the hips side to side.

7.   Keep the elbows wide.

8.   Practice control by holding each twist for a moment.

9.   Hug the knees in to the chest for a stretch when finished.

SWAN

Swan counteracts my hunchy shoulders after a big climb—I think of it as the exercise that extends my wings. It strengthens the long muscles adjacent to the spine that keep the back neutral during pedaling, which helps prevent back fatigue, pain, and injury. Most of us have felt tightness in our hip flexors and upper back while riding, and swan also helps alleviate such tendencies.

1.   Lie on the mat face down with the palms directly beneath the shoulders, the elbows tucked in close to the body, and feet pointed.

2.   Squeeze the heels together, draw the navel inwards, and lengthen through the spine to lift the chest away from the mat while inhaling.

3.   Do this without using the arms to push up. Keep the feet on the mat and the legs active and straight.

4.   Once the chest is up, lift the palms from mat for a moment.

5.   Exhale and come back down. Repeat several times.

6.   Keep the back of the neck long and crease-free throughout movement.

SHOULDER BRIDGE

I couldn't live without the Shoulder Bridge. It unwinds tension in the back and strengthens the deep back muscles that are important for balance. It also engages the large muscles in the back of the legs, which can sometimes be underdeveloped in proportion to a cyclist's strong, tight quadriceps. As the buttocks and hamstrings work during Shoulder Bridge, the quadriceps will lengthen and stretch.

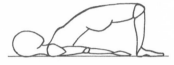

1.   Lie flat on the mat, facing up, with the knees bent and the soles of the feet placed hip-width apart, parallel to each other. Keep the arms reaching long at the sides with shoulders away from ears.

2.   Inhale, tuck the pelvis under, and slowly roll the hips up off the mat, peeling the spine one vertebra at a time away from the mat until the hips are high.

3.   Continue to press the arms down into mat.

4.   Starting from the uppermost part of the spine, roll back down with the exhalation, one vertebra at a time, until the hips arrive back on the mat.

5.   Try to maximize the breath—long inhalations and full, complete exhalations.

SIDE KICKS

I find Side Kicks deceptively difficult. They demand the integration of skills developed in the previous exercises: leg motion with a completely stable torso, strong side belly muscles, and a stable, supple back. Side Kicks also strengthen outer hip muscles that are important for keeping the knee and hip in alignment while pedaling.

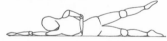

1.   Lie down on one side, lining the whole body up with the back edge of the mat. Use the bottom arm to support the head comfortably. Keep the legs straight and bring them forward at a slight angle to the torso.

2.   Lift the top leg to be level with hip and smoothly kick forward with

an inhalation, keeping the leg parallel to the ground.

3.   Glide the leg back past the line of the torso while exhaling.

4.   Keep the torso perfectly still as the leg moves through front-back motion, limiting the leg range as needed.

5.   Hips and shoulders should remain vertically stacked and square. Test

yourself by putting a hand on the hip and staying balanced.

As you do all these exercises, remember to concentrate and breathe. The next step is to integrate your newfound awareness of center with your cycling, so get on your bike, ride, and fly!

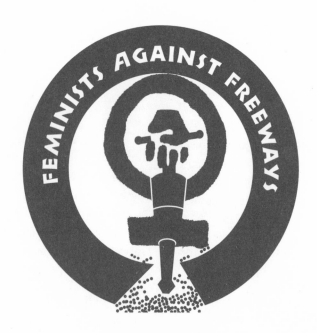

POSTLUDE

We are all trapped, in some sense, in our bodies. They are the primary way we interact with the world. They are our vessels of discomfort and embarrassment as well as our source of sublime pleasure and joy.

Being a woman in a body is a constant conundrum, because whether we try to ignore them or not our bodies have a sneaky way of meaning both more and less than we want them to. Every day when we get up and get dressed we are covering our bodies in ways that speak volumes to all we meet. Do men ponder and puzzle over their bodily functions as much as women do? Do they constantly judge every inch of the skin they are in? It's debatable, of course, but seems doubtful that they do. From the minute we are born into a woman's body we are bombarded with messages that, whether we take them in or try to leave them, suggest that we *are* our bodies. Our bodies' beauty, or lack of it, is connected and sometimes confused with our worth.

But then there's the bicycle. Truly, the bicycle is unique in its ability to make us feel and forget our bodies all at once. Riding a bike requires a body, and certain amount of anatomical coordination between brain and limbs. If you ride too long your body lets you know. Butts and backs and fingers and toes— some or all of these will tingle or tighten or throb when overused. But in between not riding and riding too long, the bike is absolutely fabulous at letting you forget all about the burden of the body. Biking on a smooth road or a twisty, wooded path, with the wind at your back and the breeze in your hair is the best antidote to civilization yet invented. We put together these essays because we wanted to dip into the vast pool of experience of women who have bodies— whatever kind of bodies they may be—and also love bikes. It's a grab bag, a grand variety, and we hope you found something you liked and saved something to come back to for another read. In the meantime, breathe deep, love your body as best you can, and go ride your bike!

CONTRIBUTORS

♥ **ADRIAN M. LIPSCOMBE** is a PhD-seeking African American mastering the world of architecture and city planning while on a bike. ♥ **ADRIANE ACKERMAN** is an unabashed rabble-rouser who's been causing a ruckus in Portland, Oregon for almost a decade. When she's not on her Cuntraption, you can find her rallying communities towards social justice, synchronized dancing with kids' bikes, and generally stickin' it to the man. ♥ **ALEX BACA** is a D.C. ex-pat working in design in San Francisco. Find her @alexbaca. ♥ **ANONYMOUS** is never just anyone, and this case is no exception. ♥ **APRIL STREETER** is the author of *Women on Wheels*, an inspiring and practical guide for city cyclists of all styles. A freelance writer, she blogs for TreeHugger and Nutcase. She is the leader of the Women on Wheels Portland riding group and the local CycloFemme events. She is currently researching and writing an historical novel about one of the first racing cyclists, Louise Armaindo. ♥ **BARB CHAMBERLAIN** is the Executive Director of Washington Bikes (WAbikes.org) and the creator of womenbikeblogs.com. Twitter: @barbchamberlain ♥ **BETH HAMON** worked for nearly two decades in the bicycle industry as a mechanic, purchaser, and shop owner. Now making her living as a singer-songwriter, Beth has produced two albums of original music and travels around the country as a Jewish music educator and cantorial soloist. (www.beth-hamon-music.com) ♥ **BIKEYFACE** is a cartoonist and painter in the Boston area. ♥ **C.E. SNOW** is a seminary dropout writing about religion, sex, and bicycling. Her first memoir, *Friction & Momentum*, is forthcoming from Microsom. Twitter: @Books_and_Velo ♥ **CAROLINE PAQUETTE** (@littlepackage) retired from an eight-year medical-surgical nursing career in 2009 and also spent eight years making cycling caps under the name Little Package. She left Portland in 2013 for the vagabond/trail/van life. ♥ **CECILY WALKER** is on Twitter as @skeskali ♥ **CHELLE D** and her dog Charlie are traveling, hiking, and biking pals currently getting things done in the PNW. ♥ **CONSTANCE WINTERS** is a freelance writer, photographer, and author of the Lovely Bicycle blog. She has recently relocated from Boston to rural Northern Ireland. ♥ **DENA FERRARA DRISCOLL** is a family biking advocate, Ikea shopper, and Development Director at a non-profit playground in the city of Philadelphia, where she lives with her husband and children. Twitter: @bikemamadelphia ♥ **ELLY BLUE** is a writer and feminist bicycle book publisher who lives in Portland, Oregon when she is not traveling to talk about bikes and books. She is the author of *Bikenomics* and *Everyday Bicycling*. Twitter: @ellyblue ♥ **EMILY JUNE STREET** is a Pilates instructor and the author of *The Velocipede Races* (Microcosm, Spring 2016). Social media: @emilyjunestreet emilyjunestreet.wordpress.com) ♥ **HALLEY WEAVER** is a slightly off-kilter epileptic cyclist from the Pacific Northwest. Blog: bikeleptic.com ♥ **HEIDI GUENIN** likes to work on transportation/land use/public health/social justice policy and play with yarn, food, friends, and bikes. ♥ **HOLLY KVALHEIM** is from Seattle and enjoys bikes, drawing, and drawing bikes. ♥ **JACQUELINE (JACKIE) A. GROSS** lives and rides with her partner in Oakland, CA. When she's not writing, Jackie can be found on Twitter (@ladyjax) expounding on life, fandom, and the general state of the world. ♥ **JANET LAFLEUR** is a Silicon Valley marketing professional, bicycling advocate, and blogger at One Woman, Many Bicycles, and founder of Bike to Shop Day. ♥ **JAYMI THARP** did not provide a bio, so we will just say that we are thrilled to feature her work. ♥ **JOSIE SMITH** works at a bike shop and loves riding the local mountain bike trails. Follow her at josiebikelife.com ♥ **JULIE GOURINCHAS** is a twenty-two-year-old college junior who likes wolves and feminism a bit too much. ♥ **K.I. HOPE** says: I aimed for your heart and missed. thegreatinanition.org ♥ **KATE BERUBE** is a children's book creator who lives in Portland, Oregon. She is the author and illustrator of *Hannah and Sugar* (Abrams, 2016), and has illustrated *The Summer Nick Taught His Cats to Read* by Curtis Manley (Simon & Schuster, 2016) and *My Little Half Moon* by Douglas Todd Jennerich (Putnam,

2016). Find her online at kateberube.com ♥ Out of all the hats she has worn, **KATHLEEN YOUELL** likes Family Biking Activist on Twitter (@kyouell), Facebook (PDX Cargo Bike Gang), and her neglected blog (portlandize.com) the best, despite the lack of pay. ♥ **KATIE MONROE** is a bike advocate and community builder in the great city of Philadelphia. She refers you to bikeleague.org to learn more about the Girl Scout bike patch program. Twitter/Instagram: @cmon_roe ♥ **KATIE PROCTOR** is a technology consultant who enjoys the bikey life in Portland, Oregon with her two children and their many imaginary friends. She has directed Kidical Mass PDX since 2010. ♥ Though you'll only ever get to meet one of them, **KATURA REYNOLDS** is nonetheless a mother of three. She rides her bike around Portland, Oregon and tweets at @katura_art ♥ **KEIHLY MOORE** is a designer of streets, places, and spaces. She is a weather lover, cyclist, artist, and optimist. Find her at completeblocks.com and mappingofminds.wordpress.com **KELLI REFER** lives in the Emerald City of Seattle, where she works as a bike advocate and loves bike touring where the wild roses and cedar trees grow. ♥ **KIRSTEN RUDBERG** is still eternally optimistic, racing her third cross season and having her ass handed to her on a regular basis. ♥ **KRISTIN EAGLE** is a crazy mountain biker and co-founder of Velohut.com ♥ **LINDSAY KANDRA** lives in Portland and likes to play with words, ride, climb, and have one-sided conversations with her dog. ♥ **LISA SAGRATI** is recovering from Lyme disease, but still suffers from car sickness. Her writing has appeared in Nerve, Red Savina Review, Poydras Review, and previous issues of Taking the Lane. She can be reached at Lmsagrati@gmail.com. ♥ **MATT QUEEN** is a product designer, traveler, and coffee drinker who lives in Seattle. Find him at mattqueen.com ♥ In June 2014, **MONICA CHRISTOFILI**, her partner, and their two-year-old son left Portland, OR with two bicycles, one baby seat, one baby trailer, and one gear trailer to move by bike tour to live closer to family in NH, and while the Pacific Northwest is now far away, the bicycle love it gave her is not; she still commutes by bike out on the East Coast. Reach her at monica.christofili@pcc.edu ♥ **NATHAN EZEKIEL** is a mid-30s white trans guy living in Cambridge, MA. He and his wife, Angela Gail, have been blogging about carfree family living (carfreecambridge) and queer parenting (firsttimesecondtime. com) since 2008. His writing also appears in the collection *Manning Up: Transsexual Men on Finding Brotherhood, Family & Themselves* by Transgress Press. ♥ **NICKEY ROBARE** is a feminist, cyclist, seamstress, and lover of sequins working in community media in Minneapolis, MN. ♥ **PARISA EMAM** is a mental health therapist and writer from Seattle, WA. ♥ **RACHEL HORN** is a cyclist, feminist, environmentalist, activist, and foodie from Los Angeles, CA ♥ **REB ROWE** is an urban planner, illustrator and steed-junkie from Adelaide, Australia. ♥ **REBECCA (BEC) RINDLER** writes, lives, and bikes in New York City. (becrindler.tumblr.com) Social media: @becrindler ♥ **RHIENNA RENÉE GUEDRY** is a Louisiana-born Leo, a DJ, and a curator of the best Halloween parties this side of the Mason-Dixon. ♥ **SAMANTHA BRENNAN** is a cyclist, a feminist, and a philosophy professor. She blogs at Fit is a Feminist Issue (fitisafeministissue.com), the Feminist Philosophers blog (feministphilosophers. wordpress.com), and her own web page (samjaneb.tumblr.com). Twitter: @SamJaneB ♥ **SARAH REBELLOSO MCCULLOUGH** is a cultural scholar and biciculturist living in California. sarahmccphd.com ♥ **SUSANNE WRIGHT** is a lover of books, bikes, and beer. ♥ **SUZI HUNT** is a sixty-eight year old, car free, wife/mom/grandma/great grandma, who re-discovered bike riding in her fifties and who hopes to inspire others to ride. ♥ **SYNTHIA NICOLE** likes quiet time listening to records & reading. She loves strolls along the creek with dogs. Find her online at zinewiki.com/Damaged_Mentality ♥ **W.D. SMITH** rides and sells bicycles in Chicago. He draws, paints and doodles in his spare time. Billy.dwight.smith@gmail.com